How To Get the Healthy Back In Your Hair

Rekindling healthy hair

By
Angela Hughes Brown

AuthorHouse™
1663 Liberty Drive
Bloomington, IN 47403
www.authorhouse.com
Phone: 1-800-839-8640

First published by AuthorHouse 10/27/2009

ISBN: 978-0-9839116-1-6

Library of Congress Control Number: 2009910319

Printed in the United States of America
Bloomington, Indiana

This book is printed on acid-free paper.

Dedicated

To

Perry C. Brown

My

Soul Mate

I

Love you Poppy!

Special Thanks...

God, thank you for loving and carrying me when I needed spiritual guidance. I can do nothing without you. You have constantly shown me favor!

Crystal Howard, you're my girl, client, and friend. I love your Christian spirit! Stay in love with life.

Yolonda Rockett, thanks for editing my book and being a supportive sister. You always have believed in me, and you have taken out the time to show it!

Lauri Deener, Thank you for pulling off a difficult job, as an editor you always capture the true message. Your support means so much to me, and congrats on your movies, and other personal projects. I look forward to watching your vision on the BIG SCREEN!

Jasmine Deener, thanks for all the help in proof reading, your future is bright, and you have grown into a beautiful flower.

Jeremy Martin, you're my oldest nephew who has just graduated let the world be your oyster. Keep God first and anything is possible!

To all my clients, thank you for supporting me through the years. You have no idea how much I love you all. God gave me the anointed hands, and you all trusted me to grow your hair. This would not be possible without you, my soul lights up with each visit you take with me. Many friendships have been born between us. I am the most blessed hair stylist in the world! Take a bow we are making history together, and you all unselfishly are sharing me with the world! All that you know about your hair, the world will have the pleasure to read for themselves. You truly know how to leave my chair and let your hair blow in the wind!

Dear Readers,

I want to encourage you to try some of my hair tips. Your hair deserves the very best. Why spend hundreds of dollars on your wardrobe, and barely anything on your hair? I urge you to read my book and understand the possibilities your hair can achieve. My book will teach you how to work with your hair stylist, and how to select a good one.

I've been a licensed beautician for nineteen years, and I've enjoyed my entire career! My clients and I connect through our minds, bodies, and souls. I have consulted with each client to understand their goals and I know their textures. Through the years, I have built a clientele that consist of old and new friends, as well as family. My formula is a two-month system that promotes hair growth, manageability, volume, and an overall healthy appearance. As a hair stylist I hold no secrets, only the facts.

Everyone was born with virgin healthy hair; however, over the years damage may have occurred. It possibly resulted from a bad trip to the salon, or your lack of understanding hair textures. I encourage you to use professional products only. Why gamble with generic products that may not have all the high quality agents your hair needs?

Read my entire book, and see if you feel the same about your hair. Your hair is alive so let it breath, and flow in the wind. I hope my book gives you vital information that will be easy for you to understand. I want you to enjoy your new hair care experience! I will leave you with a poem that is dedicated to you. Its purpose is to put you in the mood to change your way of thinking, to a positive image.

Blowing in the Wind

Take me to a jazzy place where I can move to the beat of my glory. Smooth, silky, and flowing in the wind. Never mind my ego I have earned it honey. Roll out the red carpet it is my time to shine to the fresh scent of my hair. Woo that jazz is my beat, my blues, my la cream. I feel sexy so free to be me, trumpet blow your horns, let the doves fly across the sky to witness a parade of soul. My hair is sexy, sassy, healthy, and loving me. So follow me into the clouds of love and experience your hair blowing in the wind....

Angela H. Brown

CONTENTS

INTRODUCTION
GETTING THE HEALTHY BACK IN YOUR HAIR AND CHOOSING A STYLIST

THE TRIP TO THE salon should be a wonderful experience! Your hair care should be the main reason you decide to patronize your stylist. However, there may be other reasons. Here are the main reasons people decide to stay with their stylist.

1. They love the location.
2. The stylist is a relative.
3. The stylist is inexpensive.
4. They have been going for years.
5. The stylist offers some satisfaction.

The reasons above may benefit you in some way; however, the following are the best reasons for choosing a hair stylist.

+ Experience
+ Dedication to service
+ Knowledge of hair textures, products and styles

Dedication to service means offering advice, as well as, providing quality hair care. If I felt that one of my clients were making a terrible life decision I would give them advice and it would never fail that the client would come back and say the end results were my fault! I have even lost a few people from giving advice when they did not request it. Therefore, I am very careful and I listen until asked for an opinion. In addition, I remain careful when responding.

Many people, who I have serviced through the years, were looking for the same thing, hair care! Once you've decided that you want to go to a hair stylist, focus on your goal. A consultation should be first on your agenda. It will show the hair stylist just how serious you are, and it will help the two of you see eye to eye. Remember to ask questions like, "what products do you use, what are your salon hours, and have you ever worked with my hair texture before? If the stylist becomes annoyed with your probing, beware, this stylist may have something to hide!

Some hair stylists have been in the business for years, and can become cocky during the consultation. Often, stylists feel they don't have to explain their system for hair care, but keep in mind that a good stylist will remain professional during a consultation. If a stylist wants your business they should communicate honestly. **Tip:** remember hair stylists are like doctors, or attorneys, so sometimes the power of arrogance can take over. Stylists have to come back down to earth every now and then.

My book will give you some important insights on the proper salon etiquette for both the client and the hair stylist. Two wrongs never make a right. If you are being mistreated, it's best to leave. Of course, if you want to return, air out your opinion in private; never in front of others, it only makes the situation worse!

I have shared several things to consider as you begin your journey selecting your stylist and putting the healthy back into your hair. There is one last thing to consider;

"HOW MUCH WILL MY HAIR COST? " How much is very important, you need to know if you can afford to sit in the chair! Some clients think every hair stylist should charge the same. Lose that way of thinking right now! Some clients have a problem with cost. At the same time, the proper etiquette is for the hair stylists to give their new clients a quote in the beginning. I have been in trouble with new clients before, regarding cost. Chapter one is very important to me because the client, as well, as the hair stylist need to have a good understanding. Throughout the book you will have many hot topics concerning hair issues as well as hair tips; my goal is to educate the client and the hair stylist.

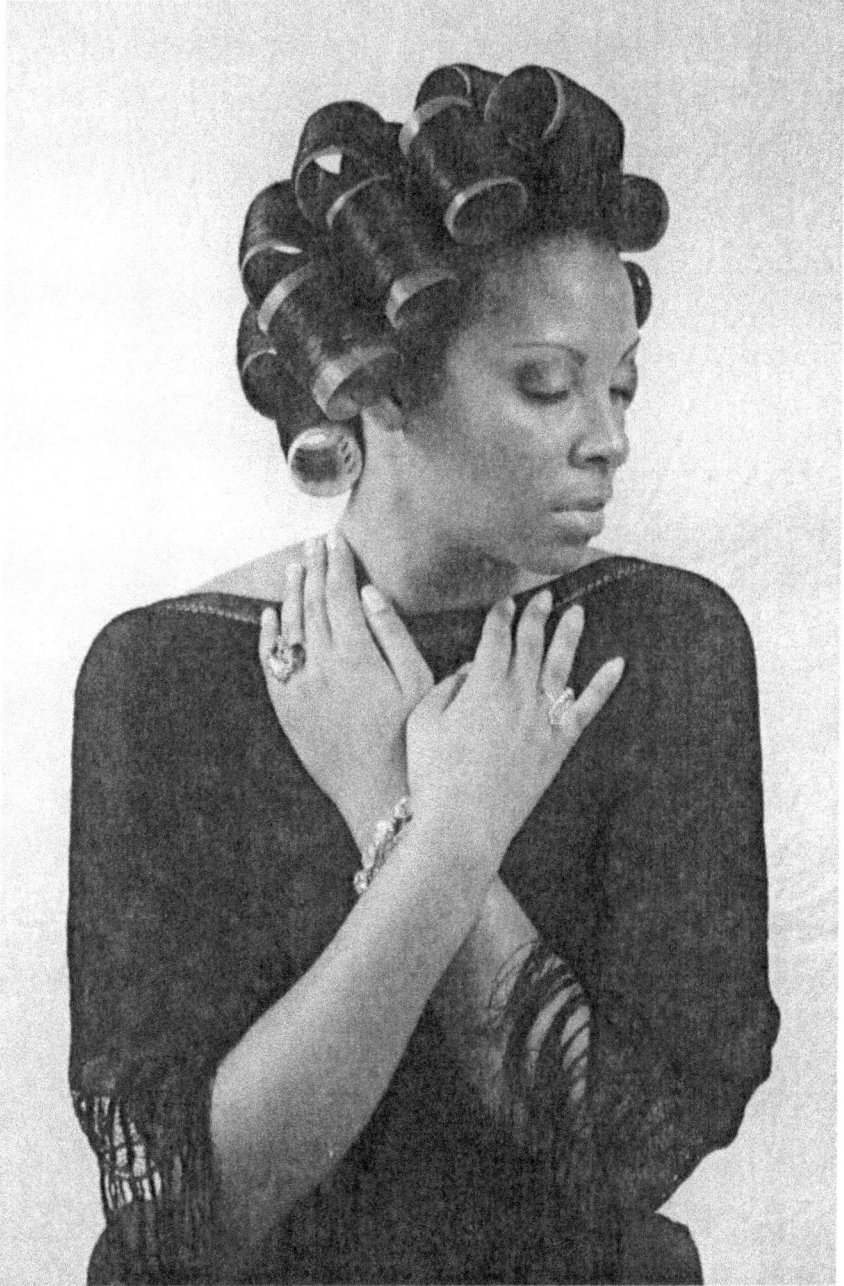

My passion for hair care will explode in each and every one of the chapters and I hope you will enjoy this up close and personal moment of my hair career experience.

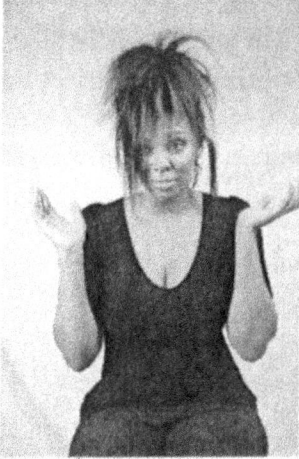

CHAPTER ONE
THE CONSULTATION

IT IS A GOOD idea to request a consultation prior to your first visit with a new hair stylist. This allows you and the new stylist to meet and greet, in addition to assuring that the two of you are a good fit. Here are some things to discuss during your consultation: 1) your hair concerns and goals, 2) products, 3) appointment time, 4) hair technique, 5) salon rules 6) hair expense and payment options, 7) health issues and allergies, and 8) vacation times.

HAIR CONCERNS AND GOALS:

Set realistic goals for your hair. If you have thin brittle hair and your desire is to have thickness and volume, remember that this may take time; therefore, have some patience. Products high in protein will aid in achieving more volume, but also be sure to inquire about products that can be used at home to compliment the products used in the salon. Be honest about your concerns. Tell your stylist if you are taking different medications. Some medications can slow down the hair growth process and a good stylist will research to find a solution to overcome your hair concerns.

PRODUCTS:

There are many products on the market, some of which may not agree with your hair texture. It is important to let your stylist know what products you are using at home. A good stylist will let you know exactly what is best for your hair texture and will provide the products for you to purchase at the salon, or tell you where such products can be purchased. Again, for maintenance, you will want to use the same products your stylist uses on your hair to obtain maximum results. Professional products are more expensive then products found at your local drug store; however, focus on your goal and understand that it may require some sacrifice in order to achieve it.

APPOINTMENT TIMES:

Appointment times are crucial to providing quality service. If one client is late, it can throw the entire day off. No one likes to sit and wait, nor should any client feel that their time is being rushed. Each client deserves quality time with the stylist; therefore, if you are going to be late, phone your stylist to see if you can be rescheduled at a later time to accommodate everyone. Keep in mind that a professional stylist has an obligation to their clients which requires them to honor the same appointment times. If your stylist is constantly late, you should have a second consultation to reiterate your expectations, and make sure your stylist can accommodate your schedule.

HAIR TECHNIQUE:

All styles are not meant for everyone. Some textures will not cooperate with every style. If you find a style that you want, ask your stylist if it is possible for you to wear a particular style. Don't become defensive when your stylist is honest with you and responds with, this style is all wrong for you. Ask what could be done to help you achieve something similar. Sometimes weaves, lots of holding spray, or just a creative stylist can help you achieve the look you want. Remember to inquire and not take it personally.

SALON RULES:

Certain salons prefer that you eat in a designated area. Others prefer that you make childcare arrangements. Understand that the rules are usually designed to guarantee complete satisfaction for all clients. Rules are not meant to offend anyone. Stylists, who value their customers, will want to create a relaxing atmosphere that does not include listening to crying babies and smelling onions and garlic from the last customer's lunch. Be respectful, obey the rules and enjoy the salon experience.

Hair Expense and Payment Options:

In some salons, the stylist may have a price list for different styles. Never assume that all styles cost the same. During the consultation, inquire about styles and if there are price differences. Make sure you understand the payment options. Your new stylist may only accept cash payments, or cash and check payments only. You don't want to get to the end of service, and find out that your stylist does not accept Visa. If you need payment arrangements on your hair care, make sure that your stylist is aware and accepts the arrangement. Very few stylists offer this type of service, so do not assume your new stylist is just like your previous stylist.

Health Issues and Allergies:

If you are allergic to a certain chemical or ingredient, explain this during the consultation. People, who are allergic to peanuts, could have a life threatening reaction if peanut oil is an ingredient in a particular product. Explain to your stylist any bad reactions you have had with certain products. Health issues such as bronchitis or asthma need to be shared with your stylist to avoid a serious reaction. A simple mask or opening a window could aid in providing you with a pleasant salon experience, rather than a trip to the emergency room.

Vacation Times:

Many clients today have standard appointment times. They come at the same time every week. If you know that you take the week of your birthday off, and go to the islands, share this with your stylist. It is inconsiderate to have your stylist hold a time for you and you fail to show.

Try to write down your questions so you won't miss anything. As a new client, you may want to look at the styles of the other clients being treated by your new stylist. This will give you a direct view of what you can expect. Give your new stylist at least two months to prove themselves. Go strictly by their system just to see if it works.   You and your new stylist should have good chemistry together. If I had to describe my relationship with my clients, it would be similar to being their best boyfriend. I make sure the service is so good they know they can't get it like this ANYWHERE ELSE! When I first meet each client I find out their wants and needs. I have a smooth system, which allows them to express their expectations, without being judged. I let each client know this is their last stop, and I totally commit to them as if I only have one client. Clients can give you clues on their habits if they are relaxed, and then the therapy begins. I love what I do, so it's easy for me to listen because I am eager to solve the problem.

Let your guard down a little to open the door to communication so he or she can go to work on your hair issues. Most hair stylists want to get right to work and sometimes that can be a big mistake! I love to connect first with my clients. I've experienced that sometimes a client may not want a connection and I respect their wishes. Generally they don't stay around. Such clients are sometimes called salon shoppers. They travel from salon to salon and no one can please them on a long term basis. One year I had a client who claimed I was the best thing since sliced bread. She even asked me to let her pay for her hair the way she wanted to, and one day she left without an explanation. I had forgotten she was a traveler; she went onto the next best thing. So I consult clients, and rather they stay or not, I know within my heart I have done the professional thing for each and every one of them.

CHAPTER TWO

TEXTURES

Y**OUR HAIR HAS A** very special strength. You must tap into what your hair is capable of enduring and achieving.

+ What makes your hair grow?
+ What makes your hair break, shed, thin out, and go bald in certain spots?

Well if you don't know you may want to ask your hair stylist. Textures are very important to understand. They are: **FINE, MEDIUM FINE, MEDIMUM,** and **COURSE** hair textures. In order for your hair to reach its full potential, you must use products specifically designed for its texture. Every product doesn't work on everyone. Love your hair enough to know what works, and what doesn't work.

Fine hair is a very delicate texture. If left untreated the client can easily begin to see excessive baldness, or thinning. Too much pressure on fine hair will cause hair strands to space far apart. The scalp can show you how each strand is placed like soft mink hair. Wearing weave and braids will cause additional thinning and can lead to baldness when the hair is very fine. Fine hair needs what I call the watchful eye technique; this texture doesn't have many second chances! **Tip: Take a wet strand of your hair and see if it has elasticity by pulling it between your finger tips. If it breaks then your hair is either over processed or it might have a conditioner, or color problem. Seek a professional stylist who specializes in healthy hair care.**

I have seen seasoned women of all races who have developed baldness. Most people will tell you it comes from aging, well that might be true in some cases, but if you practice good hair habits, then you can avoid the whole myth of the getting old and bald syndrome.

Medium fine hair has been quite easy for me to treat and style throughout the years. It loves the idea of mind, body, and soul. This texture can move, and flow in the wind on a breezy day. Medium hair can carry volume and give the illusion that it is full and very healthy. Now, this texture has to be watched as well. Make sure you do not over use products such as mousse, setting lotions, and foam wrapping lotions. This texture cannot tolerate overuse of such products, as well as, avoid overusing hair gels and holding sprays. Medium hair doesn't need to be weighed down. It also does not need to engage in any weaving activities, unless it is for special occasions. On such an occasion, try to use the technique of sewing the weave into the hair rather than bonding. Medium hair yields great results when it receives deep conditioners, mask proteins, or pure proteins. Most medium hair will produce natural oils, but if not, then apply a hot oil treatment. This hair texture can easily revert to fine hair if damage occurs.

Note: Keep all textures ends clean; this keeps the hair alive, and growing.

Course hair doesn't always mean thick and unmanageable. Most moisturizers with mink oil or aloe are great for this texture. Course hair that is extremely dry cannot take a lot of pure protein. I studied an experiment and learned it is appropriate to apply protein in moderation on any hair texture.

Note: Discontinue usage of pure protein when you notice your hair is gaining strength.

Pure protein over usage can revert the hard work you have done! Be careful, and watch for any thinning in the crown, hair line, and the nape area. Course hair can break easily if alcohol products are applied to hair consistently. Alcohol will dry the hair completely out; however, it doesn't mean that you can't apply it to your styles. Whenever you notice shedding and breakage these are both red flags to discontinue usage. **Tip: For best results with course hair, a hot oil treatment is to be applied at least once a month.**

Getting a hot oil treatment regularly will wake up all the natural oils in your hair shaft. Knowing your hair texture is important because your hair is only going to respond to certain products. My advice to you is experimenting with poor products can be fatal for your hair! A tip: Try to keep shampoos and conditioners at a 4.5ph balance if possible. I have accomplished great results using the appropriate conditioners.

Many clients have encountered hair stylists that over cut the hair, and fail to provide what the client wants. Keep in mind not all stylist do the same work; find the right one that is confident when they are cutting your hair, and have a clear understanding of what you want and need. Over the years I have enjoyed styling many different textures, it's challenging yet rewarding. Textures have to be treated with the appropriate products. Hair that has experienced damage, may not exhibit the true natural texture; however, you can regain your natural texture with the proper treatments. By eliminating the choices that led to the change in your texture, such as chemical colors, weaves, braids, and over processing with perms, can allow your hair to regain the beauty and healthy texture you desire. In addition, the texture can be restored through using a great professional hair care system. My advice is to seek a professional hair stylist who specializes in your situation. Choosing to repair your hair at home may cause further hair damage.

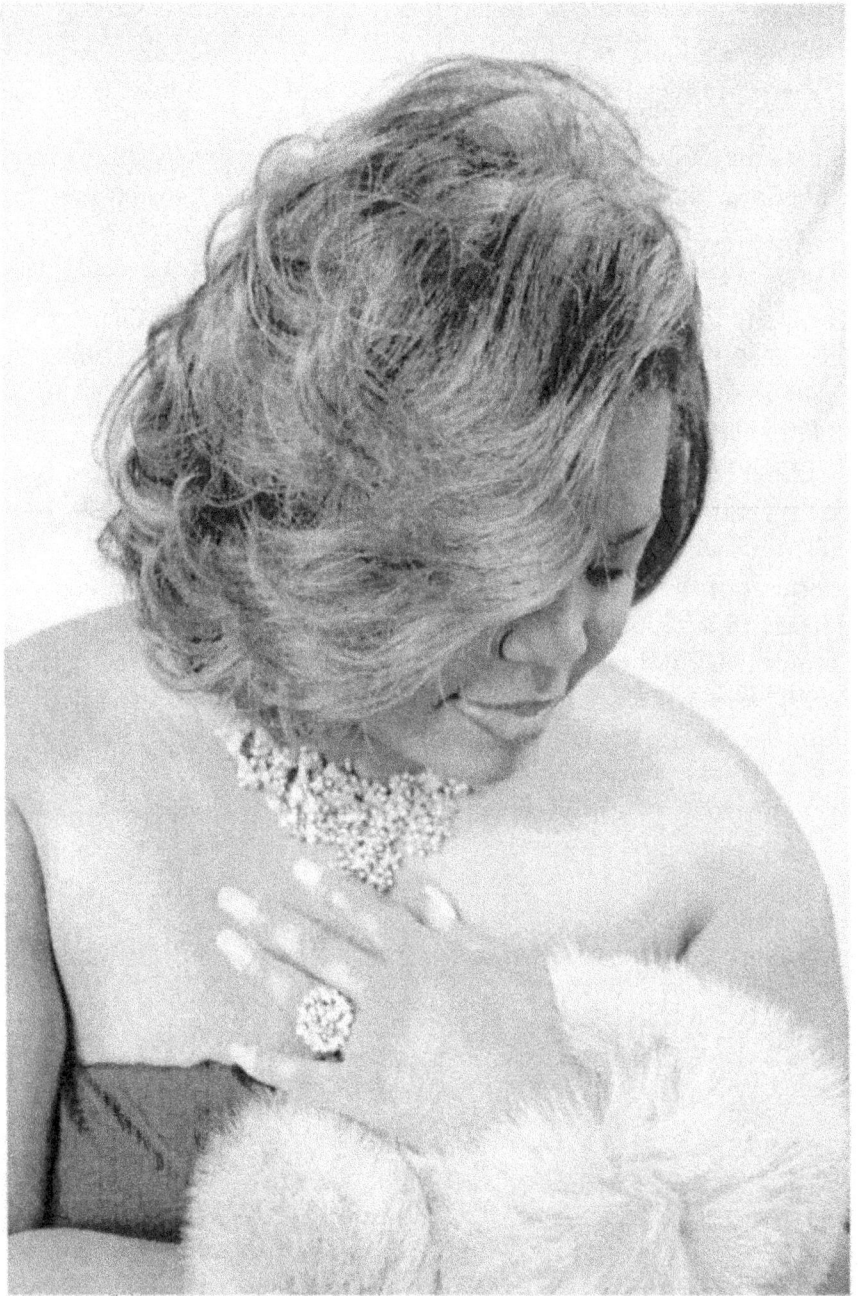

CHAPTER THREE

COLORS

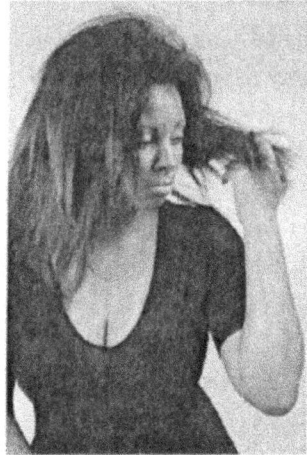

THIS IS THE MILLION dollar question, can I get a color? In my career, I have been very strict about suggesting colors. Clients sometimes need to make a cosmetic change. Choosing to get a bold hair color, can be a big devastating mistake! Make sure you get a patch test, before you change your virgin hair to color treated hair. **Note:** a patch test is only taking a few strands of your hair and applying color to the strands to test the hair; this will determine if applying the color will be a safe suggestion. There are different types of colors such as: rinse, semi-permanent, permanent, and bleaching.

Hair rinses are less damaging. They do not lift the hair; they only high light the hair's natural color. For years my clients would get a rinse and be under the impression their color was going to change dramatically. The truth is this is a non-chemical color and most rinses give you a different tone or color shade, but rarely will you see your hair lifted into a different shade. I believe rinses are safe for clients whose hair may not be strong enough for permanent colors. If you have stubborn gray hair you may need to apply a rinse when your perm has been applied. The hair shaft is exposed, and you will have more time to enjoy the color until your next perm, or relaxer. Rinses only last four to six weeks. If your hair receives the rinse, then you have a longer time to enjoy the product. **Tip:** I am using a product for the hair and scalp and this product line has a shampoo and conditioner that by experience, has given my clients a longer time before the color separates from the hair. The shampoo is called Cleanser and the conditioner is Scalp Therapy. This product line has a glycol-color shield.

Semi-permanent colors last longer than rinses and are less damaging then permanent colors. Generally a semi-permanent color will last six to eight shampoos or more and are available in gels, crèmes, liquids or mousses. A semi-permanent color is made up of pigments deposited in the hair cuticle and outer cortex that will fade with each shampoo. Many clients use semi-permanent hair color to enhance or deepen the natural hair color.

Permanent hair colors last 28 shampoos or more and penetrate deep into the hair shaft. Clients with stubborn gray hair often prefer a permanent hair color. When using a permanent hair color, keep in mind that it is indeed permanent and very difficult to change without stripping, which is harmful to the hair. Permanent hair colors have a developer and alkalizing ingredient, which serves the purpose of raising the cuticle of the hair fiber in order that the tint will penetrate, as well as it facilitates the formation of tints within the hair fiber, bringing about the lightening action of the peroxide. This is a very intense method for coloring hair and has many disadvantages. It is always best to have a professional hair stylist color treat your hair as many individuals suffer skin discolorations, irritations and over processed hair when performed at home. Over processed hair becomes dry, rough and fragile, thus leading to breakage.

Unlike permanent hair color, with bleaching, instead of depositing a color into the hair shaft, the bleaching agent penetrates the shaft and disperses the color molecules that are already there. The more color molecules dispersed, the lighter the hair becomes, thus the lighter you take the hair from its natural color, the more damage will occur. Bleaching is a very harsh process and can cause severe damage to the hair if not performed by a professional. Most colors will go inert after 30 minutes; however, with bleaching, it will remain active as long as the hair has moisture and the longer it processes, the more damage it does to the hair.

Have you ever heard the term, "BLONDES HAVE MORE FUN?" Well maybe with the guys, but if you color your hair blonde and your hair is too weak for the color, well that is not what I consider fun! Never use a high peroxide volume that will cause the hair to lose its strength.

I suggest using a ten or twenty volume; the thirty or forty volume is too risky to control the hair. **Note:** Long term usage of color is not suggested; because when it is time to apply your perm or relaxer the hair doesn't have time to repair itself. You should try to space the two chemicals at least two weeks apart. It is a good idea to write down the dates of when you received each chemical. Remember to go to one hair professional so when questions arise, you and the stylist will know the total process used, and it will be less difficult to trace the mistake.

There are different ways to apply color: frosting, streaking, and hair lightening. Frosting, streaking, and high lightening can be damaging and I suggest you see a color specialist or a professional stylist who has attended color classes and understands the anatomy of hair. Frosting gives a light effect all over the hair. In frosting tiny strands of hair are lightened to blend in with the darker hair. With streaking, bleach is applied to one to four strands of hair around the face. Lighteners can be used all over or in various parts of the hair. I never apply color to hair that is weak or too thin. Some clients may prefer their hair to be lighter in certain areas and darker in other areas of their hair. This technique is called high lighting. Always apply a conditioner to the hair after all color treatments. Your conditioner must have protein in it, or use a re-constructor conditioner. You should use a hair masque to go through the hair shaft, and repair any parts of the hair that might be damaged.

I love conditioners that have a moisturizer base; the hair can be restored if natural moisture has been taken from the hair. Remember the hair is weakest when it is wet so use a large rat tail comb to detangle the hair. Larger combs are safer, because smaller combs tend to pull the hair out when it is wet.

You should never perm, or relax the hair the same day you color the hair unless it is a rinse. You might as well get ready for a cute wig because you will be wearing one until your hair grows back.

One day I had a client suggest that I damaged her hair, and I was appalled because I had not seen her in months. I knew she would occasionally treat her own hair, and would see two other hair stylists including myself! I just listened and professionally explained my views. Once I finished talking to her, she was not at all concerned about solving the problem. I have learned it is very hard to properly give your advice if you have a bossy client who has no clue how their hair care system works.

Clients who feel they know more about hair than the stylist sometimes can cause a problem. They have a deaf ear to any suggestion. My advice is for such clients to stay out of the salons and consider doing their own hair at home.

I love the idea of color if applied properly, but the nightmare enters when a client's hair can't take the chemical, and when the hair is already damaged.

Chapter Four
Relaxer, Is It For Me?

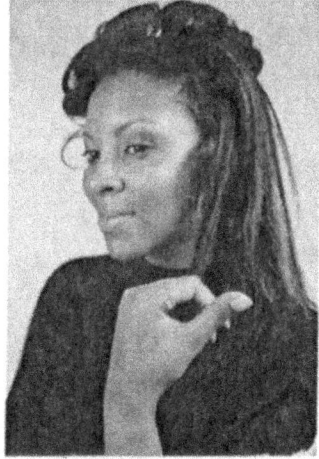

RELAXER IS A COMPLEX chemical, it can make you gorgeous or your hair extremely damaged. I never use the same relaxer system on each client. Clients need to feel they can trust you and you won't damage their hair. Relaxers come in different chemical forms lye, and no-lye. The term relaxer means to relax, and some clients and hair stylists want to over straighten their hair. African American people generally can use relaxers when they are trying to straighten their hair. Caucasians can also use the relaxer system depending on if they have very curly, kinky hair textures. Caucasians or any other nationality may use the term perm, which is used to curl the hair. Both can be damaging if not applied according to the professional standards. Never assume you can perm or relax your own hair. Your hair does not deserve that kind of abuse. When applying the relaxer use a fine tooth comb to assist you and ensuring you don't over process the hair.

No-lye relaxers are for clients who have sensitive scalps. For clients who have color, fine texture, and scalp issues, the no-lye relaxer system really works best. You should apply this relaxer to the most sensitive areas last. I have seen clients who have experienced severe blisters and soars from applying the relaxer wrong. Remember to base the scalp thoroughly before applying the relaxer.

I always give my clients a protector cream. This is applied through their hair and it blocks the relaxer from overlapping into the hair that doesn't need relaxing. Your hair over a period of time will be over processed, and will need extra hair care. This can be very costly. If you're not a professional then you should never apply your own relaxer

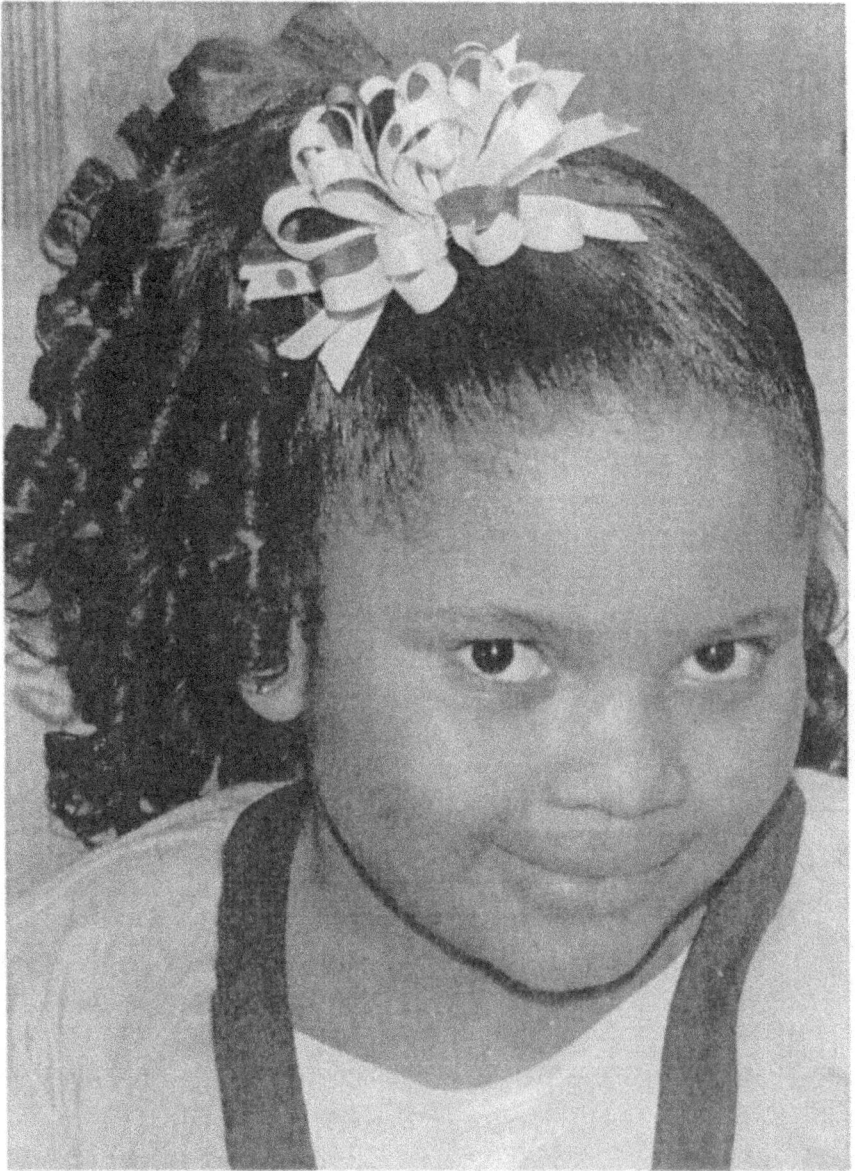

It's difficult for you to see your entire head and successfully escape from damaging your hair. Ask yourself is it worth the risk of damaging or losing your hair?

Sodium relaxer is just your lye relaxer that usually breaks down a little faster and can burn if you do not base the scalp. You technically do not use this relaxer on color treated, fine texture, damaged hair, and naturally curly hair. This relaxer can thin the hair faster and you cannot out work this chemical. **Tip:** When trying a new stylist remember to give the stylist a heads up on what relaxer works and what doesn't work for you. Be persistent because your hair should be top priority. From my past experience, I studied relaxers that have conditioners in them that have worked well for me and my clients. Some relaxers can leave the hair feeling too dry; meaning the natural oils have been taken out. **Tip:** Never get a relaxer and color chemical at the same time. You might as well get in line with your former pictures. That means pictures you previously took when your hair was long, thick, healthy, bouncy, and just gorgeous. I suggest you space the two chemicals at least two to three weeks apart. My clients usually wait three weeks, and I always prepare their hair by applying re-constructor conditioners.

I have to clear up all the questions about my children who are on their way to experience the world of chemicals. Moms, I suggest you do not allow your little angels to get a relaxer under the age of four. By the age of five it might be up for question if the hair is easy to revert back and pressing the hair is a waste of time. You can consider a texturizer. It is a little less harsh and you may experience better control when you comb and style your child's hair. Chemicals are a big responsibility, so if you're not going to commit to bringing your little angel to the salon, then leave the chemical alone until you are really ready. Children should have a chance to let their hair fully develop and if the chemical is not applied correctly then the hair cannot truly reach its natural growth. Make sure your child's first relaxer experience is at the salon, and use a no-lye relaxer. The no-lye has to mix and the stylist can control the amount your child might need. If your child is getting a relaxer and she burns easily, then the relaxer should be applied to the sensitive areas last, to avoid irritation. **Tip:** If your child is very young then try not to apply the relaxer to her edges first. Leave the baby hair alone if she doesn't have a kinky wave. If your child has deep wavy hair then I suggest the texturizer to loosen the

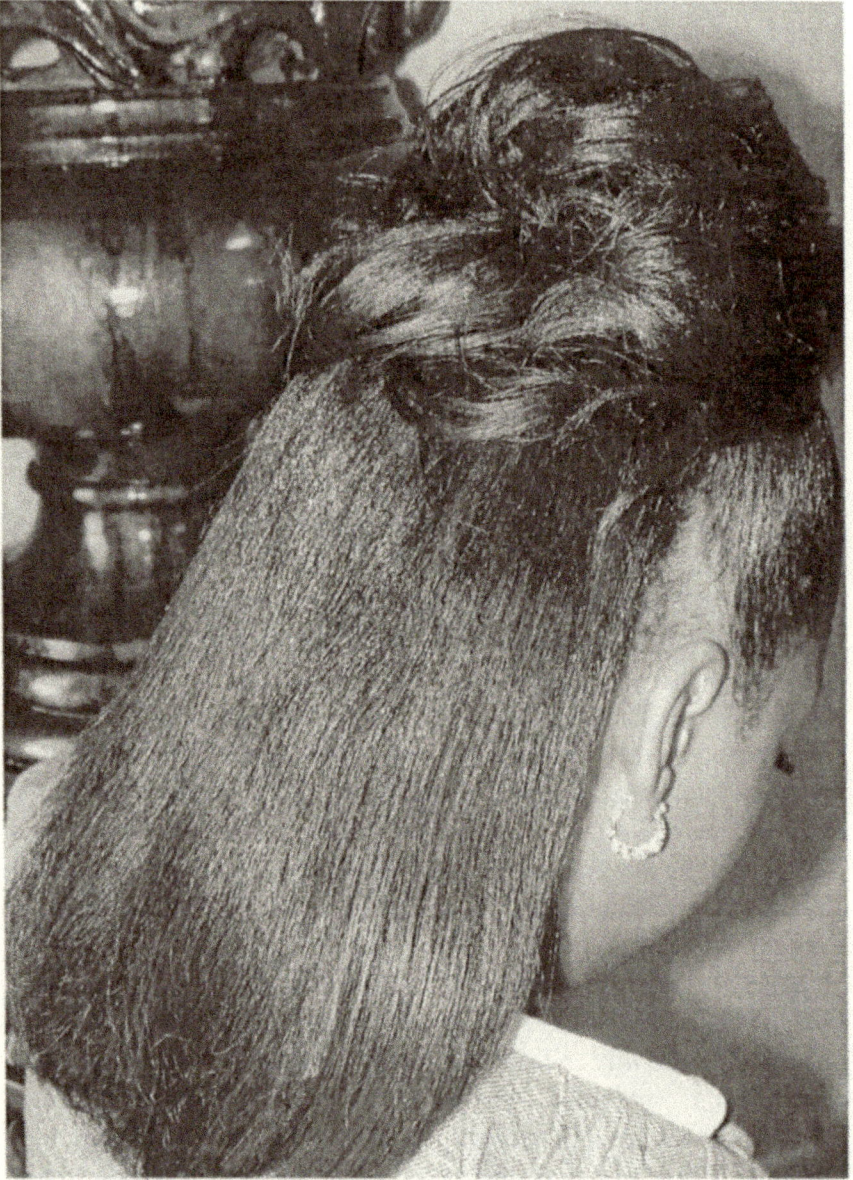

wave but allow the natural wave to return when it is wet. The child can wear curly or straight styles. **Tip:** If your child swims then make sure you shampoo the chlorine out with one neutralizer, moisturizer shampoo, and conditioner. The relaxer in their hair can't take the chlorine and it can cause damage.

Clients who have medical issues with their scalp may not want to get a relaxer; it could worsen the condition in the scalp. Solve the medical issues first then consider the chemical, and consult the dermatologist on your plans regarding the chemical. A Nioxin hair and scalp specialist, and the owner of Concept 2000 beauty and barbering, Alberta Nibley remarked, "You can tell what drugs and medication a client may be taking and the color of the drug or medicine will show up while getting a relaxer." Gold is an indication of antibiotics; green is a warning of marijuana; purple is a sign of high blood pressure or cocaine. Some drugs weaken the hair and can cause a negative reaction with certain chemicals. For this reason, it is vitally important that you discuss your medication with your hair stylist to avoid a chemical reaction or hair loss. Also read the prescription warnings conveniently located on the prescription bag, and question your stylist to make sure the products used in the salon do not contain any ingredients that could cause side effects with your medication.

Clients who are getting perms or body waves should make sure they use a professional product first. Perms can be damaging if not applied properly. Perms can be used on hair that is straight in texture or that has a natural wave. These clients are trying to get their hair to curl and have volume. Clients have to shampoo the hair first then go into the system. You must roll the hair on end papers and use perm rods. Make sure you time this process to keep from over processing the hair. If there are any straight ends the hair might be over processed and the stylist will have to clip the ends. Usually with a perm, the client does not shampoo the hair for a couple of days to allow the curls to set in.

The perm and relaxer system can be a wonderful process but a professional should be the one who performs the treatment. **Tip:** When you have a client with two different hair textures then you can apply two different relaxers to keep the other texture from becoming damaged. African Americans can have many different hair textures. Usually I try to analyze their hair texture. If the entire head has not reverted back at the same time, then you can apply a partial perm. A partial perm is defined as, relaxing half of the client's head and the other half at a later date.

Some clients only need a texturizer. This is a chemical that will make the hair curl. If applied properly then the client can wear their hair curly, or straight. If a client feels that they aren't quite ready for a relaxer then this is best for them. Press and curls sometimes can be a waste for clients especially if they tend to sweat heavily. All chemicals can be successful if applied properly. Make sure you neutralize the hair each time twice after each chemical. Texturizer's can be styled best with a moisturizing lotion, that dries with a vibrate shine. You can also style with mousse, setting lotion, and hair glossifier. Soft & Beautiful Botanicals, has a great texturizer, with natural plant extracts. Botanicals, is formulated to enhance the natural wave and curl pattern, developed to protect hair and scalp during the texturizing process. This process leaves the hair soft, curly and natural looking. You can achieve various hair styles curly wet, dry set, body wraps, two strand twists, and much more!

Kimberly Williams Greer, a professional hairstylist of over 20 years, and personal hairstylist for Gina Neely of the Food Network Show, *Down Home with the Neely's*, and *Road Tasted with the Neely's* recommends that clients commit to regular salon visits when deciding on relaxing their hair. Kimberly stated, "Your life style determines if a relaxer really is for you. With relaxer comes commitment. The commitment is to become knowledgeable, about your hair texture and type." Consulting with your professional stylist is your first step. Knowing what type of commitment you're willing to make when it comes to salon visits and maintenance is important to promoting healthy hair, she added.

CHAPTER 5

INTERMISSON

A LITTLE SHOP TALK

A WOMAN WALKED INTO THE salon on a Wednesday, she had no appointment but insisted I style her hair. She called herself Katrina, darling. Oh my goodness she kept referring to herself as Katrina, darling. I introduced myself as Mrs. Kathy Turner the owner of Healthy Hair. I'm the proud wife of Mr. Thomas Turner the owner and top chef of Miami's number one restaurant Cherry Wine. Luckily I wasn't busy so she sat in my chair and took off her $1,200 laced wig, and dandruff flew everywhere. I noticed she wore over $100,000 worth of diamonds on her ears, hands, and neck. Amazingly I could estimate that her hair would potentially total at least $250. If hair could be on crack then consider her hair addictive. I began small talk as I started to my magic. I asked her had she had the pleasure of tasting the rich food and desserts at Cherry Wine Restaurant. She actually had gone there because a friend referred her and told her it was the most happening "hot spot". I blushed because she shared with me that she thoroughly enjoyed her meal, the service and her whole experience.

She looked at me slightly different, but from her body language I knew she was in no mood for small talk. Ok back to business, I escorted her to the shampoo bowl, and placed the towel and cape on her. My shampoo bowls recline back and your feet are elevated upright. The water hose has a jet spa experience. I love to massage the client while shampooing because it relaxes them and Ms. Katrina seemed to be calming down.   Oh my Lord! Hair was shedding everywhere. I asked her if she was aware of the hair loss. Her response was, that is the reason for the wig. I explained the need to apply a protein to help reduce the shedding. She opened her eyes and asked me to do my best and to leave out all the gory details. I went straight to work. First, I applied the pure protein, and added the re-constructor conditioner that has a balance of moisturizers, vitamins and controlling agents that will slow up the shedding. I love to use the two products together because it has a way of tightening the hair shaft and I also use a scalp shampoo called the cleanser that goes underneath the scalp and repairs the hair follicles. Mixing conditioners

Can be very good because one does one thing while the other takes care of another.

Katrina spent only twenty minutes under the dryer for her conditioners. I used a ph balance of only 5.5 or 5.6 to lather her hair and restore lost natural oils. Katrina's hair began to wake up, the Paul Mitchell Tea Tree cleansed her scalp and removed the dandruff and left her scalp feeling refreshed.

The last phase was to cut her hair. Katrina had shoulder length hair and an oval shape face. One of the main reasons for the cut was her hair was too thin and she looked like the old man in the Poltergeist Movie where he was trying to get the little blonde girl named Caroline to follow him into the light. So I was destined to bring Katrina into the light and let her scalp breathe from that wig.

She was on the prowl again she looked in the mirror and pulled her hair in disgust and fell back into the chair and said, "Have your way honey, I am your guinea pig, but make me look human." The loud mouth all of a sudden had no words. Was the world coming to an end? I prayed and went to work I had a wonderful cut in mind, it was a razor cut mini bob. I cut the front with my shears to have thicker weight and I gave her swoop bangs with layers. Then I angled the bob in 90 degree angle and gave the crown 40 degree layers and increased in angels as I went down to the nap area. I razor cut the nap area to give it a softer texture. Her cut was almost complete so I left her sides a little longer with full layers to give her body and movement. I set the hair with alcohol free mousse and a leave-in conditioner. I placed jumbo rollers at the top and medium in the middle and back. Katrina was placed under the dryer for a few minutes because she had no patience. I blow dried the rest of her hair, beveled her hair with a flat iron and gave her a few feathered flips. I took the cape off and turned Katrina to the mirror and she let out a loud scream. I jumped and asked her if she was alright? She said, "No, no, please don't get me wrong, I love it! My hair looks great!" Katrina hugged me and when she finished hugging me I clapped for her.

She began putting on her makeup and she cleaned up well. She never needed that wig. I explained to her how she needs to remember she should treat her hair just as good as her clothes and jewelry. Now here was her first step to not being cheap with her hair, I gave her the bill for today. "Katrina your total for today is $210.00". She gave me a fifty dollar tip I knew she would be back. Katrina could not stop looking in the mirror all the way out the door. I gave her my business card and she left.

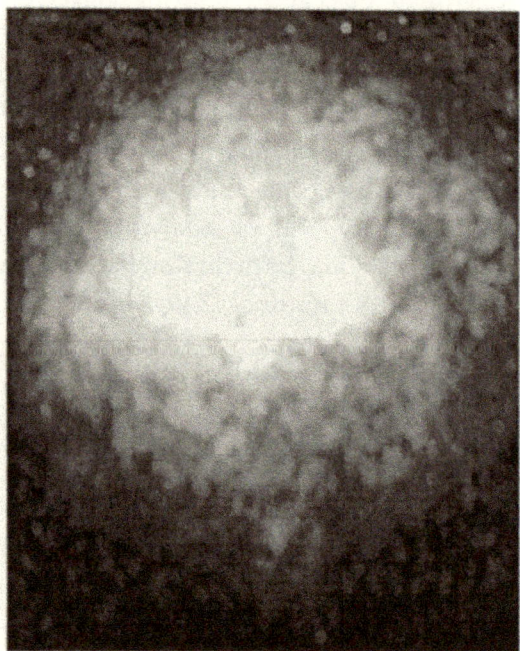

CHAPTER SIX
TOO MUCH HEAT!

Now you may ask the question "Am I putting too much heat on my hair?" Well nine times out of ten if you have to ask then you just might be putting too much heat on your hair. I educate my clients on how not to put too much heat on their hair. I provide them with hair tips that will allow them to continue to have healthy hair. Heat can be very dangerous because it can cause long term damage. Place a hair strand on a white towel and look closely at the thickness when hair is damaged. Pull the strand and if it snaps then your hair shaft is damaged. Using heat three times a week or more is too much. Example, when you use the curling iron on a daily basis the hair has already started to accumulate dust particles and the products are now starting to remove themselves. If you look at the curling iron you will notice the iron has a collection of dirt and build up. Over a period of time you will notice that the texture of your hair will start to look and feel different. Your hair will become dry, brittle, split, and thin looking. Sometimes the hair will have an unpleasant odor if you are applying too much heat. Here's a tip: When you have messed up your hair overnight, you can get a glass of warm water and take your finger tip and put the warm water on the middle of your hair. Try not to place the water near your root or scalp area. Water can revert the hair near the scalp. Roll the hair tightly from the bottom to the scalp. Please do not use any mousse or setting lotion if you want body restored. Walk around the house allowing 15 or 20 minutes and that curl will be restored. If you need extra hold then use the mousse or setting lotion. This system has worked on my clients for years.

Steam can also be damaging so try to place a satin bunny cap with the shower cap on and when you have finished showering, remove the shower cap first and wait a few minutes. Next, remove the satin bunny. This allows the hair to cool and the steam to release and not destroy the hair and cause the hair to lose the curl. Now steam can be good if the hair is rolled. The steam can reset the hair if the hair is tied down or covered. Excessive heat is extremely damaging. Everyone is different, and if you have a very busy life then try to use my tips or develop your own with little or no heat involved. Heat can also put a terrible odor in your hair. Dirt will build up on the curling iron, and that goes right into your hair shaft causing damage. Putting too much heat on your hair is an easy fix in today's world; everyone is in a big hurry! Try my water system and good rolling skills. Love your hair enough not to develop this dirty habit.

CHAPTER SEVEN
STRESS IN MY HAIR

I'VE HEARD MANY CLIENTS ask, "Why is my hair shedding?" Sometimes stress can play a big factor. Some clients have so much stress in their lives until it causes stress in their hair. The affects of stress are sometimes so extreme until the client can experience baldness. The spots are attacked usually at the crown, front, and nap areas. If left untreated, this can cause the hair to thin all over. Using protein conditioners, hot oils, and scalp treatments definitely can cease this from rapidly spreading, but the stress has to be resolved. When these treatments fail you may have to consult a physician, or dermatologist. I had a client who received needle shots in the scalp area where the baldness existed.

If you are a client and you use weave parts such as pony tails, or wig lets, make sure you give your hair a break from time to time to prevent the hair from stressing out and thinning. Weave, if worn for a long period can leave the hair very stressed and unhealthy. Braids can stress the hair out if not done properly. Some braiders can carefully make sure they follow the right technique, but some stylist or bootleggers have little concern. Using glue to braid the hair is very unhealthy! Stylists like me have to work too hard to get the clients hair healthy again.

I have seen professional braiders who take pride in their work, the finished product is beautiful, and the client can get hooked from the look. What looks good is not always what your hair needs. After the braids have been taken down I have noticed a lot of stress on the hair. If not taken down properly the hair can become thin or the scalp can suffer severe permanent damage. You cannot continue bad hair habits and expect great results.

The way you roll your hair can also be stressful; the tension you apply can be too much for the hair. Rollers that have the comb teeth sometimes pull the hair causing the hair to thin out. Foam rollers if used need end papers to prevent the hair from being pulled on the side of the roller. I often refer my clients to use the old school method, and my suggestion is to pen curl the hair. You can pen curl the hair around the outer parts of the hair. If you are wearing a body wrap then this technique will still give you body and control. Rollers with the clamps can put a crease on your hair if you do not know how to properly roll your hair. Switch the pattern of how you roll your hair. If you constantly use the same format then the hair gets used to the partings, and you can form a permanent part in your hair. It is very important to use good healthy hair care tips at home; this makes it easy for your hair stylist to perform better behind the chair.

Your personal life can hold a vital impact on your hair and scalp. Mental and physical stress is very stressful on the hair, as mentioned in the beginning chapter. Remember whatever is causing you to stress needs some attention as soon as possible! The scalp and hair will suffer greatly if that is the place where the stress will invade. I have seen many cases where clients have suffered from baldness, and extreme shedding. Some issues arise with an irritating itchy scalp. Psoriasis can occur on the scalp and it will have to be treated by a dermatologist, or hair stylist who has expertise on the subject matter. Many people hide their pain, and in some form it will come to the surface. For nineteen years I have studied the human hair and scalp, and it has been a challenging experience. I love what I do and hair is a subject that always has room for improvement.

BE WEAVE IT OR NOT

Weaves have taken new heights, and this has turned into a million dollar hair styling business! Everyone is either wearing a weave, wig, or some kind of hair piece. You may not wear it everyday, but you may try it at some point in your life. I love styling healthy hair, but every now and then a client will ask for a weave. Weave can be stressful on the hair. My advice is to make sure that the process doesn't result in hair loss. If at anytime I feel that a client is wearing the weave too long then as a professional she will no longer receive that service from me. Here are a few different types of weaves that clients may ask for:

1. Bonding
2. Infusion
3. Lace wigs
4. quick weaves
5. pony tails
6. Sewing
7. Braiding
8. Dreads
9. Twist
10. Hair clips

Some weaves are simply not healthy for the hair. There are people who think wearing a weave will actually grow their hair. Below is a list of reasons why people will wear a weave in their life time.

1. New look
2. Loss of hair
3. Celebrity status
4. Career change
5. Curious about how long hair will look on them
6. Looking for thick hair
7. Fitness

Although weaves look fabulous, there is still a big risk if you start wearing your weave all wrong. Hair clips by far are the safest, because they can come out daily if you desire so. Sewing the weave in the hair can be safe as long as it doesn't over stay its welcome. Three to four months is too long to wear a weave. The hair needs to breathe and get the proper conditioners.

The kind of weave hair that you use has a lot to do with the out come as well. I only use 100% human hair, and I stick to only two brands. Every time a new client wanted to use a different brand there was always trouble. When you sacrifice quality weaves for cheaper weaves, you risk hair tangles, shedding, color loss, and ultimately, hair loss. Now just because the hair says 100% human hair it doesn't mean you won't have trouble! Hair that has been on the shelf too long in the beauty supply

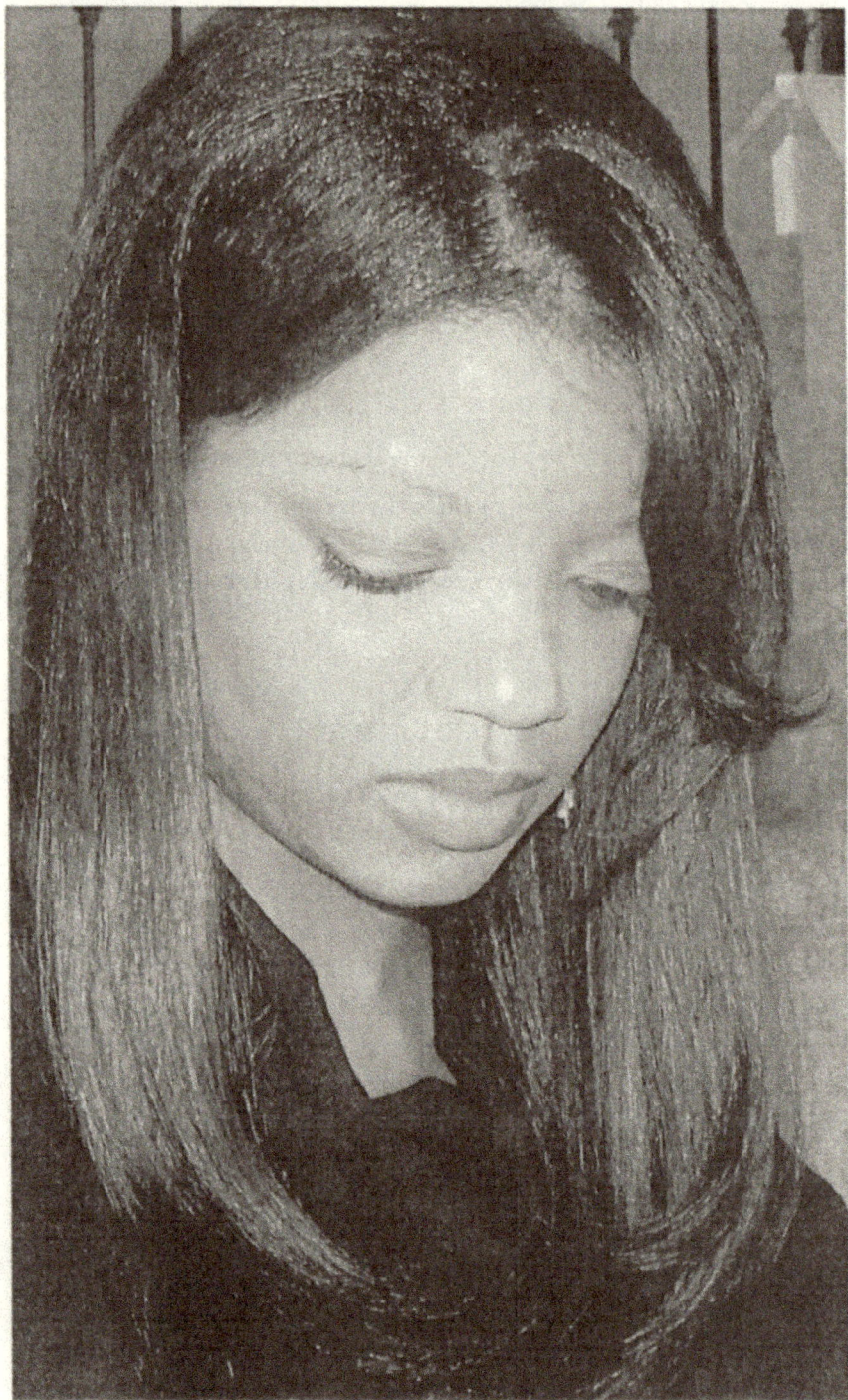

store can be a lot of trouble as well. Check out the hair first; pull it a little to see if it has loose strands. Before you use the hair, have your hair stylist clean the new hair. Remember it has traveled sometimes from other countries, and tiny micro bugs have been known to travel with the hair. The Discovery Health Channel had a segment on weave hair, and how the bugs get into the hair. Once the show ended, my career went to another level. I began to educate my clients on how to keep their weave clean. Some hair stylist style the hair after they are finished putting the weave in. This process should be avoided, because the micro bugs are virtually impossible to see with the naked eye, and can cause scalp irritation. If this occurs, the weave may have to be removed immediately and you could have to undergo scalp treatments to remove the bugs. In the event your stylist does not want to wash your weave, you may want to do so yourself to avoid a scalp infection.

Synthetic hair is for a temporary look. Many clients will want to wear it for a week or two. Synthetic weaves come in all colors and styles. It is a quick look for the client who loves spicing up their look. You cannot put heat on synthetic hair, it will burn! Never use synthetic weave for long periods. Most synthetic hair can't be combed like human hair and the styles do not last as long as human hair weave styles. Hot rollers and rods can give you a better look with synthetic weave, especially if you're wearing braids.

In addition, putting too much weave in is damaging and it only gives you a drag queen look or a French Poodle. You want to achieve balance and a natural look when selecting weave and styles. Remember the weave looks softer when your face is revealed, such as wearing the hair in a pin up style. Don't try to copy cat another person's look, get your own. Stylist should keep in mind when applying the weave on clients; make sure they can be versatile with their styles. I usually weave the hair where they can wear their hair up or in a pony tail when they work out.

The expense of wearing weaves can be costly. Generally a good bag of human hair will range from $75.00-$600.00. The more you pay for the weave, increases the length of time you are likely to tolerate wearing it. Quality weaves look more like your own hair. The cost purchasing the weave and having it put in your hair can result in you spending a few hundred dollars to perhaps over a thousand. If you pay this much then make sure the job is being done by a qualified and experienced professional. Remember the chair you choose to sit in may cause you a long term horrible experience.

There are weave experts out there who constantly practice their skills; this means they attend classes and hair shows. You can sit in their chair knowing you have to write your check out for hundreds of dollars. Infusion has become very popular as well as lace wigs. Both are performed by using glue. The infusion can be done by using wax, or the hot glue gun. This is a tedious and precise procedure. You have to apply the weave strand by strand. The process takes six to ten hours. The hair looks very much like your own and your fingers should be able to claw through your hair. The glue is twisted very refined with the weave and hair at the root.

Now the lace wig is fitted around your hair line and glued down. It looks as if the hair line is very natural. Now there are some very bad lace wigs out there; people are still thinking cheap. Whether you are wearing short or long weave, make sure it looks classy and rich. If you would like a more indebt consultation, then go to my website and purchase a consultation package, and email me with your concerns. Log on to www. thehealthyhair.com, or e-mail, angela@thehealthyhair.com.

Chapter Eight

Intermission
A Little Shop Talk

"**G**ood morning ladies and you too Chris."

"I told you miss thing my name is Christy."

"Whatever, your mama named you Chris, I love you and today we will get along, remember this is a professional environment and we do not shout all over the salon." The phone began to ring.

"Good morning, A New You Day Spa and Salon, may I help?"

There was a pause as Sharon nodded her head back and forth, suggesting yes.

"This is Mrs. Sharon Taylor and yes I am the owner. Tuesday, at one will be just fine. What service will you need? Shampoo and style, great I will see you then, bye."

Oh if you are wondering who I am, Mrs. Taylor I own the day spa, and beauty salon. I have long days and staff that are just like my own children. I work hard to keep the salon in a professional environment. They slip up at times, but they know that I do not play! Oh lord! Here comes my 9:00 she is on time as usual because I charge a 10% late fee. She is a law student, and her name is Kim, she is also a smart young lady an impulsive shopper. When she is not studying she is shopping on line.

Kim loves to wear her hair in the infusion hair weave. It is a $1,200 hair process and it blocks my entire morning, so I have to charge that amount. She loves it because it gives her the length the good Lord didn't bless her with. I think Kim believes it is her real hair because she would never be seen without her weave.

I still treat the hair with conditioners and proteins. Whenever I take the hair out, I shampoo, condition, and clip the ends properly. I let her sit under the dryer to get the excess water out of her hair, then I blow dry the rest. I bring her back to the chair to start the infusion process. During this process you must part the hair in very tiny sections, unlike how they did Britney Spears hair at the music awards show. You could see all her weave, and her bad color job! Whoever did that needs their hair license pulled and burned! Stevie Wonder could see it was a mess. Well I get the glue gun heated and I use weave that is flown in from Brazil, she has to pay for that separate, because that hair is $600.00 by itself. Once the hair comes in then the appointment is made. Kim loves the sixteen inch and she wants the long layers cut for volume. I proceed with taking small amounts of hair and squeeze the hair together and you and use tweezers to tighten the hair closely. Some beauty outlets have kits that you can buy; it has a perfect recipe for getting started.

"Kim do you like your hair," I asked?

"Now Sharon you know this is so major I love it as usual."

"I have spent over six hours, and my day is still not finished. Kim you're going to knock them dead at the all white party on Friday."

"Girl I know if this little dress I bought in New York doesn't get it then the hair will."

Kim walked out the salon and got into her black BMW, pushed the sun roof button, and checked her hair again, placed her Gucci shades on and drove off with her hair blowing in the wind. Well another one who is pleased and hair is teased.

I am so hungry, what am I going to eat? Chris, call my lunch order in at Frenchie's Quizine.

"It's Christy, Christy, is that so damn hard to remember?"

"Boy place my order, and tell them not to put so many olives on my salad, and give me extra raspberry vinaigrette."

"Ok, Mrs. Taylor, is there anything else," Chris asked, sarcastically?

"No, that is all, and thanks so much for ordering my lunch."

"Hum huh, you're welcome." Chris mumbles under his breath, "But you still need to get my name right. I don't know who she thinks she is calling a boy name when I have lipstick, and a bra on!"

Well let me get ready for my next client, she's a weave client as well, but this will be painless. This is only a sew in, and I am getting ready to shampoo her tracks. Keeping the hair sanitized is a must, because bugs and bacteria can cause the scalp to become badly damage. One day I was watching the discovery channel, and they showed how white bugs laid eggs, and hide in the weave tracks. I almost fainted, there were thousands just playing around, like it was their home. I made sure each time I would style a client's weave I vowed to never put the hair in dirty! A lot of stylists don't care, but I do. You must educate your clients about this situation. I charge so much because I am more detailed, than other hair stylists.

Well here comes my lunch, and after I eat my client will be coming in shortly. She likes her privacy because she is an actress. I'm so good, because everyone thinks it's her hair and the fact that she tells them it's hers. One day I was sick, and she was going to the Grammy's Award Show, she pulled me out of bed and tripled my money to style her hair. I felt so much better when the limo pulled up at my house, and took me to my salon so I could create a miracle at the last minute. Well here she comes again. I am going home as soon as we are finished!

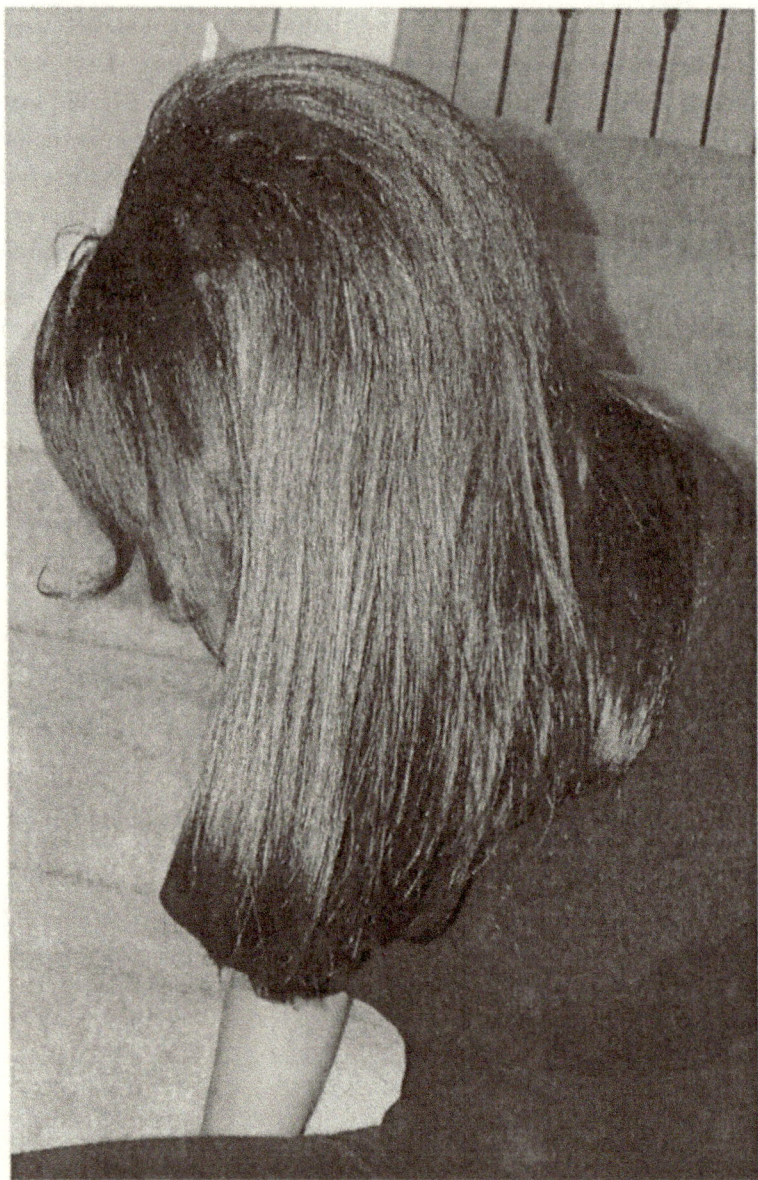

CHAPTER NINE
HELP! AM I PAYING TOO MUCH FOR MY HAIR?

OH YES THIS IS the juice that many people have asked over, and over again, "Am I paying too much?" The question is, "Are you worth it?" Some clients are willing to pay hundreds of dollars on their clothes, shoes, and little on their hair. When I first started in the business nineteen years ago, I was afraid to say how much my client hair service cost. Now, I know that I have earned the right to say what I am worth!

A worthy hair stylist uses products that contain a balance of oils, vitamins and minerals. The cost of hair care will vary from client to client depending on the current condition of the hair. A worthy stylist shops for high quality products, attends shows and seminars to learn the latest hair care products and styles. Keeping this in mind, should help you in deciding if the stylist is over charging you. When you visit a stylist and the products in the salon are what you would find at your local drug store, then you are in the wrong salon. Only stylists that have enhanced their talent and perfected their skills, have the right to be more expensive. **Tip: Ask how much the stylist plans on charging. This keeps down confusion. It also makes the visit go smoother and everyone is on the same page.**

If your friend or someone you know refers you to their stylist; it is never a good idea to compare prices, because their service may be totally different from yours. You and the hair stylist need to have a one on one consultation. The best products can be very costly and if the prices increase it is almost inevitably that the cost of your hair care will increase too. Your hair deserves the very best and you want your hair stylist to use products of quality. **Tip: Go through your financial expenses and find out what you can afford to spend on your hair. Salon owners have large expenses which may give them a reason to look at their overhead ultimately causing a cost increase.**

Location is also important; some salons can give you a fantasy of life. The atmosphere is outstanding and you may incur a slight cost for that. These salons are at your service from head to toe. You will be able to encounter these mostly in upscale beauty salons that also have a day-spa. They will greet you with spring, or bottled water. Oh yes, they are on time and they serve you only! A salon with a low overhead doesn't charge as much. It is probably in a less desirable location and the salon may need a lot of maintenance. Some stylists rarely renovate their salon and they over charge. This certainly should not be your salon of choice. Ask yourself if your hair looks rich and healthy when the wind blows. If you can't answer that question with an affirmative "yes", you're probably paying too much and your hair isn't healthy.

Clients need to be aware of the hair stylist who charges according to what the bills are. Once the bills are paid then he or she may change their fees. Sometimes they will complete your hair only when they need the money. I also need to make you aware of the stylist who charges according to how much money they think you have. You the client have a right to ask for a price list, before you venture to a new stylist. If he or she doesn't have a list then, make sure that he or she is consistent with how they charge you.

The hair industry varies from year to year; hair stylists may receive price increases from their distributors as well. This has an impact on the client also. Everything is increasing, from gas, to property value, as well as hair care products. You must consider hair stylists are their own bosses and will need to give themselves a merit increase from time to time. Like in any profession a raise must be earned. Trends can change; therefore it is customary for your stylist to keep up with the times. **Tip: Please make sure you can pay for your visit to the salon. Bouncing checks give off bad signs that you're in over your head or you're not able to manage your money effectively.**

Clients can get too comfortable and play money games. Example: Asking you to hold their check until they get paid. Clients can bounce checks and refuse to handle the situation until it's appropriate for them. In my career I was blessed to have a wonderful clientele with the exception of a few bad seeds. I have learned once I started giving certain favors I was taken advantage of. I had to learn in order to save my business I had to take charge of my business. Clients sometimes will leave you and as a professional hair stylists, I welcome that because it only weeds out the bad seeds!

Go through your budget see what is more important. If you can't afford to have cosmetic hair do's then just concentrate on hair care. Consult with your stylist and develop a system that works, and one that you can afford. Shop smart for your hair, see what you can get for your dollar. You may have to go to a salon without the fancy scenery. You may have to go every two weeks instead of every week, but when you go make it count!

Suggestions: Get your conditioners and sit under the dryer, keep your ends neat and clean, try styles that are easy to keep.

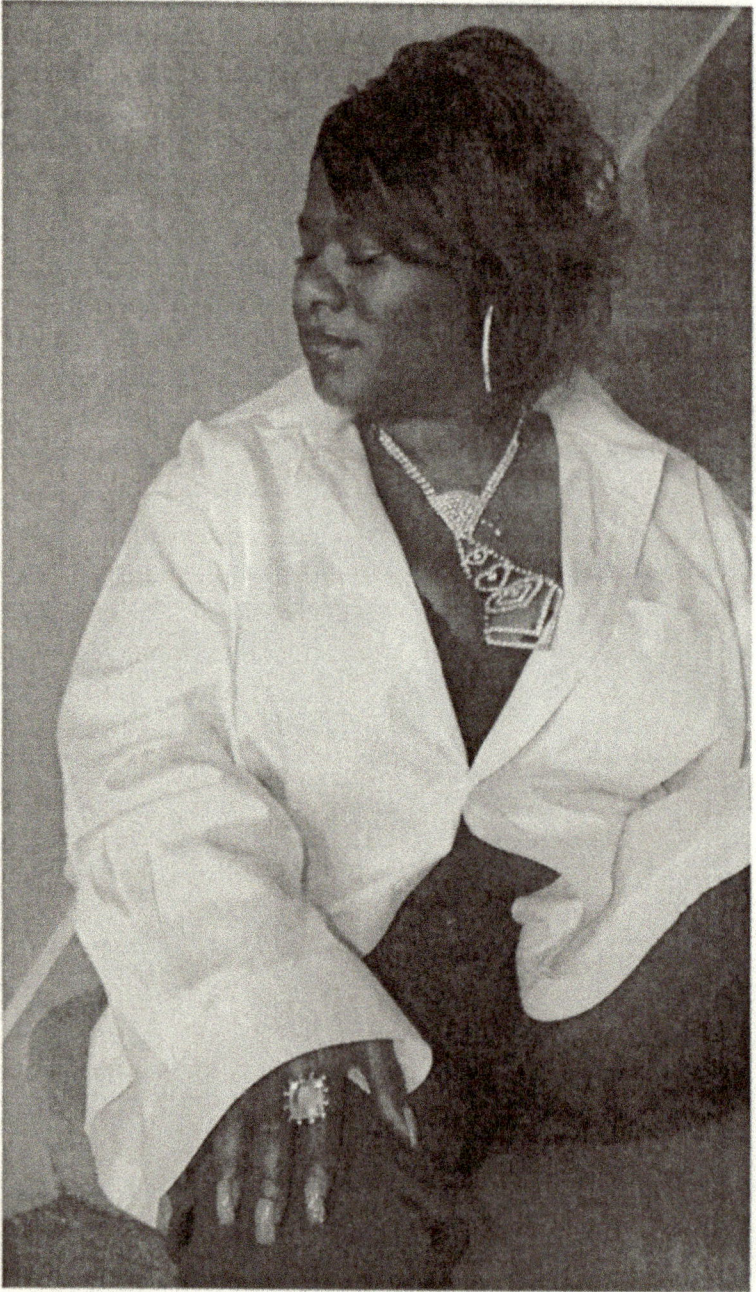

CHAPTER TEN

WHEN TO LEAVE YOUR STYLIST

I AM NOT ENCOURAGING ANYONE to leave their stylist unless your hair is starting to suffer. I have seen many stylists forfeit their skills in the hair business. They may concentrate on the financial gain and not focus on the client's needs. It is very unprofessional for a stylist to hold secrets from the clients concerning danger zones they need to be aware of! The stylist is the professional and you should attack the matter before it gets out of hand. Clients depend on us to make the right decisions, and even when a client is insisting for me to do something I know is damaging to their hair, I REFUSE! They will have to go somewhere else.

If your hair starts to lose its way then confront your stylist. If they make you feel silly or get an attitude with you, then your connection has been disconnected. Make sure you are not the guilty party, before you attack the situation. Take pictures of your hair when you start going to a new hair stylist. If your hair has begun to thin consult your stylist immediately. Ask yourself why has my stylist not said something to me? Be respectful when you question your stylist, but be stern. If you desire to give them a second chance then follow strictly by their instructions. Your hair should turn around in at least two months; if nothing is changing for the better you should leave immediately and find a hair stylist who specializes in growing hair. I call it growing hands.

Clients have often asked me to give them a color I knew would take their hair out. I can't pamper them, I have to make a professional decision and generally it is only in favor of the hair. I do not perm or relax my clients hair until their texture can and will allow it. Professionals need to get back to what is best for the clients. A stylist should clip the client's ends to prevent the hair from continuous splitting. Often a client will request to have their ends clipped. However, some stylist confuse clipping with cutting. This truly can turn off a client. As a stylist it is necessary to prove to the client that you understand the difference between the two. A good stylist will offer a hair analysis to point out exactly what needs to be clipped to provide the best results in hair growth and manageability. Both should be in agreement with the clipping suggestion, prior to the stylist beginning the process.

You may want to consider leaving your hair stylist if he or she is always running late. Please keep in mind, they are human and things do happen, but if it is a real problem, then you may have a decision to make. Hair stylists sometimes have a bad reputation on being late. I have been guilty of this in the past. I knew I would probably be there all day, and I would take my time showing up. I learned there are many hair stylists out there and I could easily be replaced. My clientele started decreasing, and I got my act together. I also realized that my clients have schedules and their time should also be valued.

Clients realize when you are not in a mood for styling their hair. You must never put that in their spirit. In this business, a stylist must arrive with a pleasant personality, and continue despite the obstacles one may encounter throughout the day. Avoid gossiping because you never know who knows who.

Your hair experience should be a great one. I love to inspire my clients. I encourage them to do well in school as well as in their careers. It is important to sow good seeds; I believe you will yield great results. You may not know it but clients see their hair stylist like their little therapists. What are you leaving your clients with when they leave? Things can get messy easy when you begin to gossip, or talk too negative. Also never give poor advice to clients, like if they should stay or leave their relationships. I lost a weekly client due to my advice. When she chose not to leave her husband, she chose to leave me. I never made that mistake again.

Putting clients in front of other clients can also be a problem. No one needs to think another client is more important than the other. I have worked with hair stylists who had no conscience about doing that. If this is being done to you then confront the stylist and see if you can resolve the matter first before considering leaving. Once you have properly spoken about the issue if things do not change you may have to leave? Sometimes a stylist needs time to grow and mature, try them again at a later date if you feel they were good at their craft.

Chair hopping can be very dangerous for your hair. I have seen clients leave stylists due to chair hopping, which means they are never satisfied with any stylist. They are always waiting for the next best thing. Some clients move for no good reason. They barely communicate with their stylist and they look for any excuse to leave the stylist. If you have hair concerns let the stylist know. If there is a new trend, you would want to try seeing if your stylist can achieve it first, before you take a flight. Hair stylists depend on you showing up its how they make a living, you should reconsider being a shop hopper. Now by all means if your hair stylist cannot deliver the styles you request, then you may have to get with a more experienced hair stylist. It is always customary to alert your stylist, especially if you have a standing appointment. By doing this the stylist can replace your appointment time with another client. I have felt the same as my clients that chose to leave. Some people are only meant to be in your life for only a season.

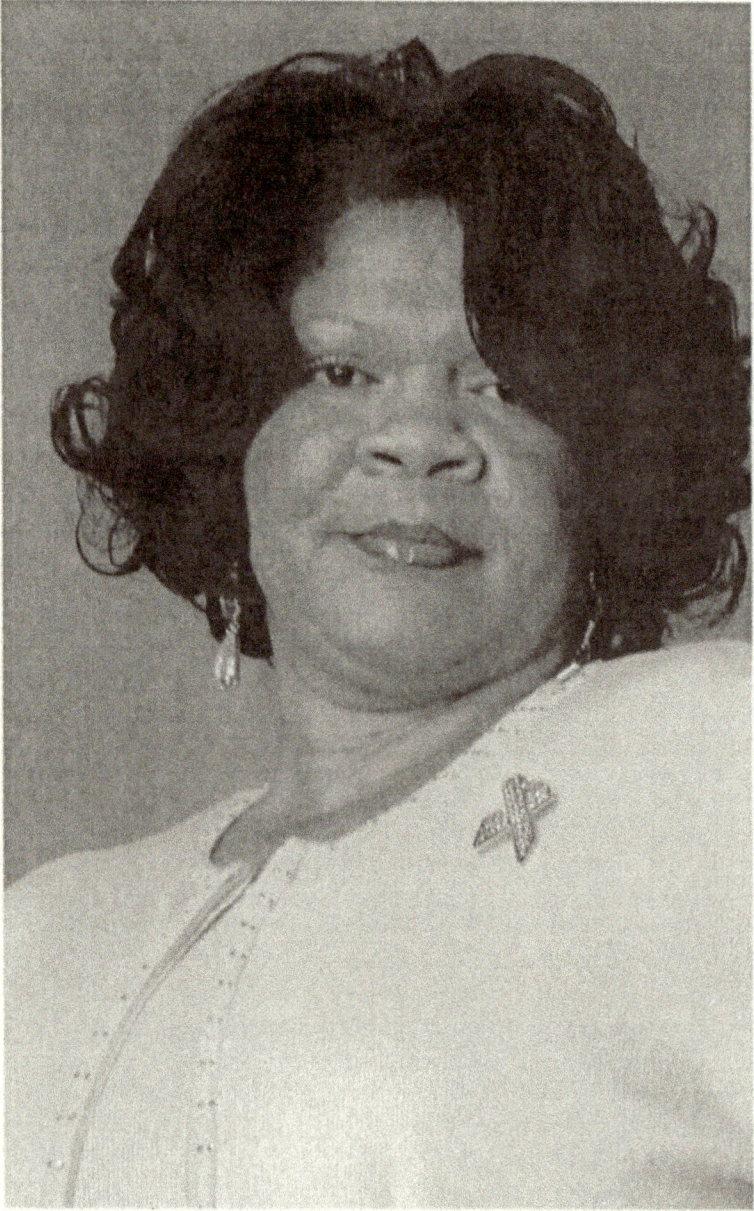

CHAPTER ELEVEN

CANCER CLIENT: CANCER SURVIVOR, MILDRED ASHFORD

MY NAME IS MILDRED Ashford. I am a two year breast cancer survivor. I have endured for over two years, many physical, emotional, and appearance changes in my life. Mid August of 2006 I was diagnosed with breast cancer. I fell to my knees and cried of having to live with the fact that my life was closing in on me. It was devastating! Being that I'm well-driven and optimistic, I refused to give up. I had to be strong for my two sons.

My sons and I talked about the cause and effects of having breast cancer and what they should soon expect. I was motivated by my sons and family not to give up. Being that my oldest son was a senior in high school and the other a rising scholar, I could not let them down. Obstacles I endured included chemotherapy, radiation, and I am presently on a medication called Tamoxifen. Soon I began regular visits to the West Clinic in Memphis, Tn. I notice my hair shedding at which time I contacted my stylist Angela H. Brown and she assured me that she would help me regain confidence in my image.

We began a regimen for scalp treatments and eight months later I begin to notice hair growth and a different diva within. Being consistent with my hair care treatments after being diagnosed with a medical condition, resulted in my hair returning more lengthier and I have found self-fulfillment thanks to God and secondly Angela H Brown.

Wearing your new hat with Cancer

As a hair stylist, hearing the traumatic news that a client has cancer, poses a new way of approaching different hair styles. As we know the chemotherapy and radiation treatments will likely take the hair out at the root. Any cancer patient will tell you that losing your hair is one of the most painful experiences. If you are a cancer survivor, try the following suggestions to help you regain your confidence.

+ Pray for direction on your hair journey.
+ Prepare yourself mentally for hair loss.
+ Have a private conversation with your hair stylist and alert them of your situation.
+ Know that your stylist is a professional and sensitive to your hair lose.
+ Take a close family member or a friend to purchase at least two wigs and make it a fun experience. Remember, laughter is the key to recovery.
+ Bring your new fun hat (wigs) with you and make an early appointment for privacy.
+ Always leave one wig with the stylist to keep clean and prepare for your next visit.
+ Continue to pamper yourself at all times with make-up, manicures and pedicures.
+ Once your treatments are over it's time to get the healthy back in your hair. Advise your stylist that you are in remission.
+ Massaging the scalp during the shampoo and hot oil treatments will loosen the scalp, stimulate growth, and keep it from drying out.
+ Keeping a short hair cut is necessary until the hair begins to grow.
+ Continue shampooing and conditioning with a hair mask.
+ Once daily use a natural vitamin oil to penetrate the scalp. Make sure you rub it into the hair evenly.

Chapter Twelve

Up Close And Personal
Hair Care Advice

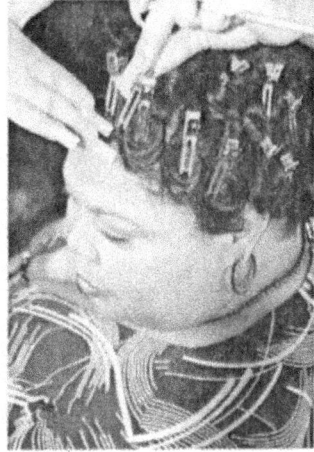

NOW THAT I HAVE opened the door to my world of dos, and don'ts, concerning hair care, I want to share some more information with you. First of all, I strongly encourage you to purchase professional products. I have used a variety of professional product lines. I stayed with one particular product for a long time, because you know the saying, "If it isn't broke, don't fix it." Another popular product line has a wonderful tea tree shampoo that acts well as dandruff and itchy scalp treatment shampoo. There is another product that has a power house protein treatment that will decrease hair shedding. You have to be careful because pure protein can be dangerous if not used properly. My number one product that I use has a 5 in1 conditioner that I will always live by. It reacts as a deep conditioner as well as a re-constructor. You can sit at the shampoo bowl or under the hair dryer.

I have a two month system that has worked for years. First, I provide a consultation. During the consultation, I write down my concerns as well as the client's concerns. Secondly, I begin my special report; each client has his or her own system I feel everyone has different issues so why do the same system that may not be effective. Once I have confirmed that we are in agreement, I then discuss a price. Clients sometimes have to budget for their hair; therefore, I try to avoid surprises. My formula for healthy hair usually consists of a cut, or in-depth ends clipped. I then move to a hot oil treatment, conditioner, or protein treatment. I also recommend at home professional

products. This is a necessity in order to achieve maximum results in healthy hair. If the client has extreme issues then I use a popular new product that has a follicle booster that is great for thinning edges, nap area, or the crown. Those are very popular areas for women, yet for men, it is generally the entire crown extending to the front of the hair line.

I also recommend rinses. If the client has a bad color the rinse can act as an umbrella to cover and protect the hair. If the client has extremely dry hair the rinse can block the sun from continuing to damage the hair. I follow up with a strand test, and I may even take photos to see how the progress is coming along. During this process I never do any permanent colors because this only slows down hair growth. Clients hate this, but in the end they love the idea! If the client has a relaxer or perm, it is best to suspend their chemical for a short time, if the stylist feels their hair has been over processed. Within two months I have always seen great improvement. Now that's how to get the healthy back in your hair!

You may have noticed America is on a weight loss kick, and the hair sometimes suffers. It is important to remember the hair can become damaged if you don't take care of it while you're working out and dieting. Extreme dieting where you go without food for long periods of time and especially purging will increase hair loss and may change the texture when dieting be aware that the hair needs nutrients to thrive. A multi vitamin can replace nutrients lost when you are reducing your food intake. Nioxin Intensive Therapy Multi Vitamin is high in marine concentrate which helps to promote strong, healthy hair. In addition, health stores provide vitamins especially for the hair, and can also be used in place of a multi vitamin. To lose weight and maintain a healthy body, skin and hair, remember to decrease your fat and meat portions, while increasing fruits, vegetables, and dry beans for protein.

Keep your hair deep conditioned, and once a month make sure you hot oil your scalp. Natural oils can escape from your hair shaft. Hot oils will replace the missing oils. When working out make sure you try not to exercise with your hair down, the sweat will go through and make your hair lose its body. Up hair styles really can work if you sweat excessively. A body wrap is fine only if it is hard for you to break a sweat. You can pin your hair around and let the sweat escape from your hair before you try to comb out your style. You may have to increase your salon visits to make sure your hair is staying healthy according to your diet. Many clients feel it can be a waste of money to travel to the salon. Try to go to the salon the day after your last work out day. Keep your forehead clean because the products will sweat down on the skin, and it may cause irritation, or fine little pimples. Only try to go to the steam room when it is the last day before your visit to the salon. If you shampoo your hair before you go then you may put your conditioner on your hair, and massage it in with your hands and the steam will deep condition your hair.

Braids can help as well only if you plan on a hard work out. I recommend braiding your hair with medium or large braids; this is for short term use only. Try not to get addicted to the braids, because they can be damaging if not put in properly. In order to maintain healthy hair, never wear braids for more than a month.

It is not beneficial to color hair, if it has been damaged. Color only makes things worse; it speeds up the thinning process. **Tip:** Take a mirror and look towards the back of your hair to see if your hair looks thin. If it does, you may need to reconsider getting your hair colored. You may have to just settle for a rinse instead. **Tip:** If you use a black brown or ash tone rinse color in your hair, put a small drop of red in the color and mix it in, gently. This is not to change the color you desire, it only makes the color look enhanced and rich, as well as it decreases your chances of getting a green cast.

I want to give the seasoned clients some hope before hair shedding starts. Now there is an awful myth out there about mature clients losing their hair, because they have matured in age. Some cases have been that mature clients may be on medication or may not be able to travel to the salon. Now I have mature clients, and their hair is very healthy. I keep their hair in good condition. Some stylists are not very patient with the more seasoned clients, because they can't sit very long. Well one scalp treatment I use has great products that hair stylist can apply at the shampoo bowl, and get the same effect that you would get if you were under the dryer. In short, the myth is not true, the only thing that has been verified is that the older you get the slower your hair will bounce back from horrible damaging circumstances.

Procrastination is also another way to destroy the hair, if you or your stylist have discovered that your hair is damaged then you must react as

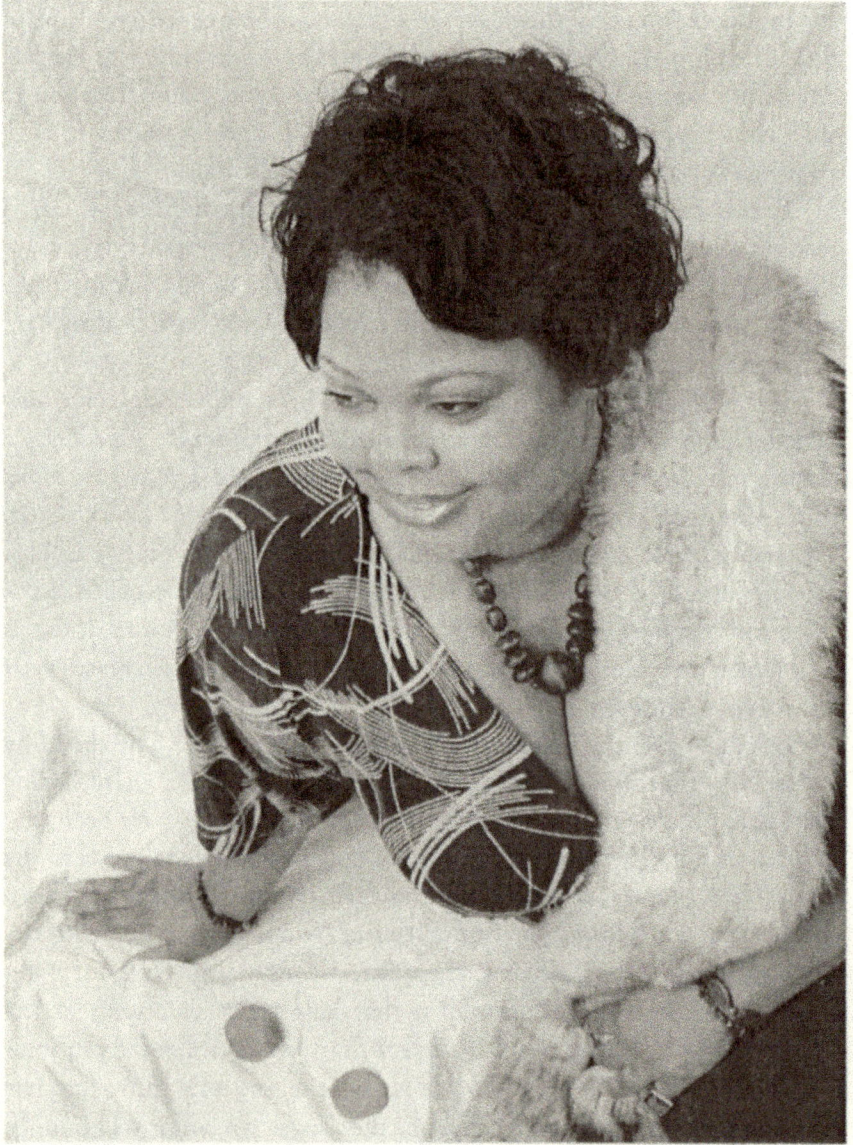

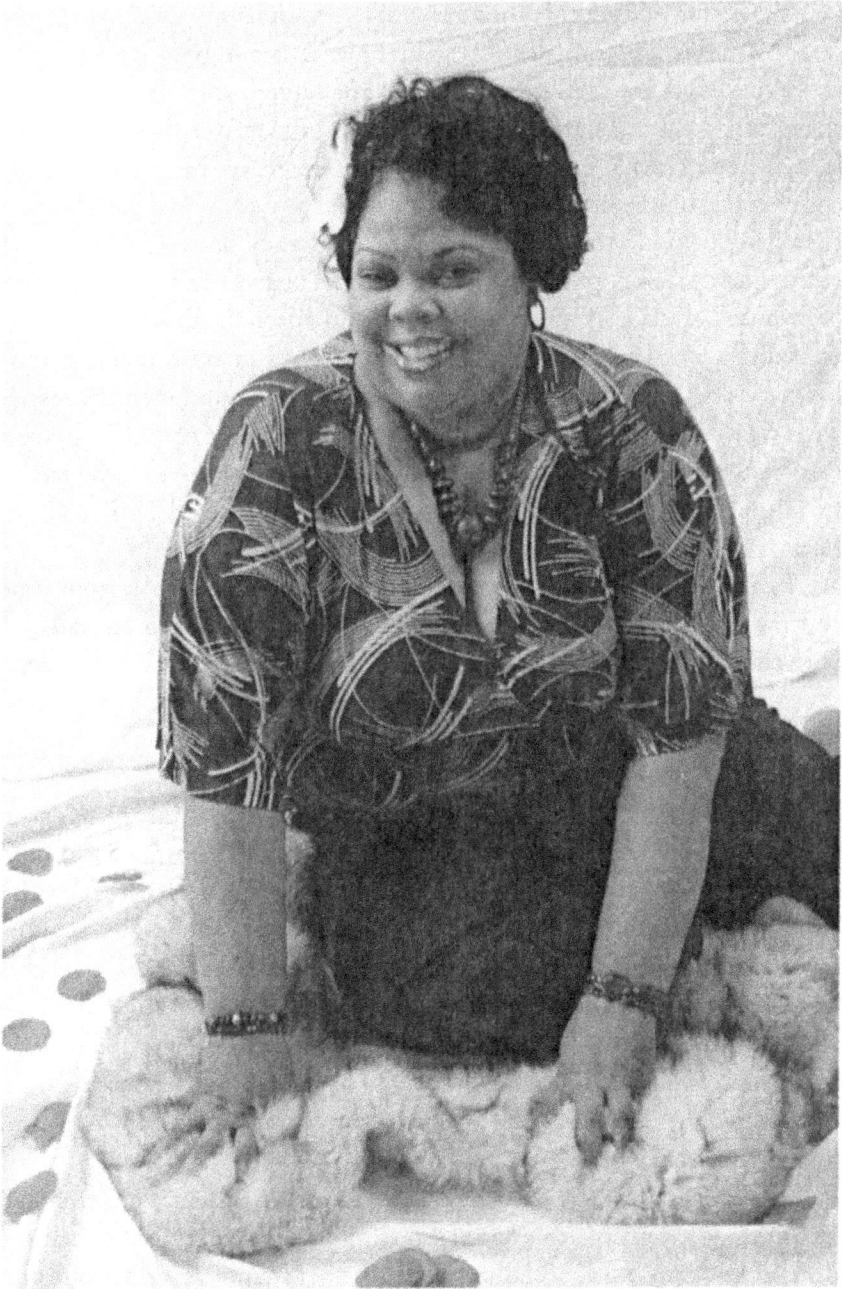

soon as possible! Procrastinating is only making your recovery process more challenging.

Now I am ending this chapter with the number one hat that client's wear that has and can destroy your hair. It is the wig, weave, pony tail pieces, and wig lets. Now don't get me wrong you can wear one of these hair pieces or hats, but let's be practical you were not born with it so let your glory breathe from time to time. Weave can enhance your appearance, but if you are reading this book, and you want healthy hair then I'm speaking to you! If your hair is already damaged the weave reacts like a leach, it pulls and tugs until it has conquered and taken out every weak strand. Wigs smother the scalp and hair. Example: If your outdoors lawn is green except were the garbage can exist, imagine your hair reacting the same way with a wig. Hair is alive and it can't breathe with weave and wigs on top of the hair. Now I admit that I have worn weave myself and braids, but my hair fell out and it took years to recover from that nightmare! That is how my journey began and I just want to help the world get the healthy back in their hair!

Be the diva and wear your hats, but give your hair a break from time to time. I have seen clients run out of money and have to cut corners with their spending. When they take the weave out, the hair is damaged causing embarrassment, thus leading to the client going back to wearing the weave. This is due to a lack of patience in waiting on the hair to improve.

Your hair is your glory given to you by God, and somewhere down the line you lost your way. I even pray for my client's hair, we ask God for everything else so why not ask him to bring the healthy back? Get to know your hair, meet every strand for the very first time. As hair stylists we are smart, but it also helps for the client to cooperate with us as well. Now on the other hand there are some stylists who do not care about their clients. I feel that they need their license revoked, but they are the masters in the business, they eat, breathe, and bathe hair. I have to toot my horn, because if I don't know anything else I know hair, and love every strand.

Well that's what you need, a stylist who will go the extra mile for you. I encourage my clients to learn the technique of their stylist. Smell the different shampoos, especially those that are unfamiliar, and inquire.

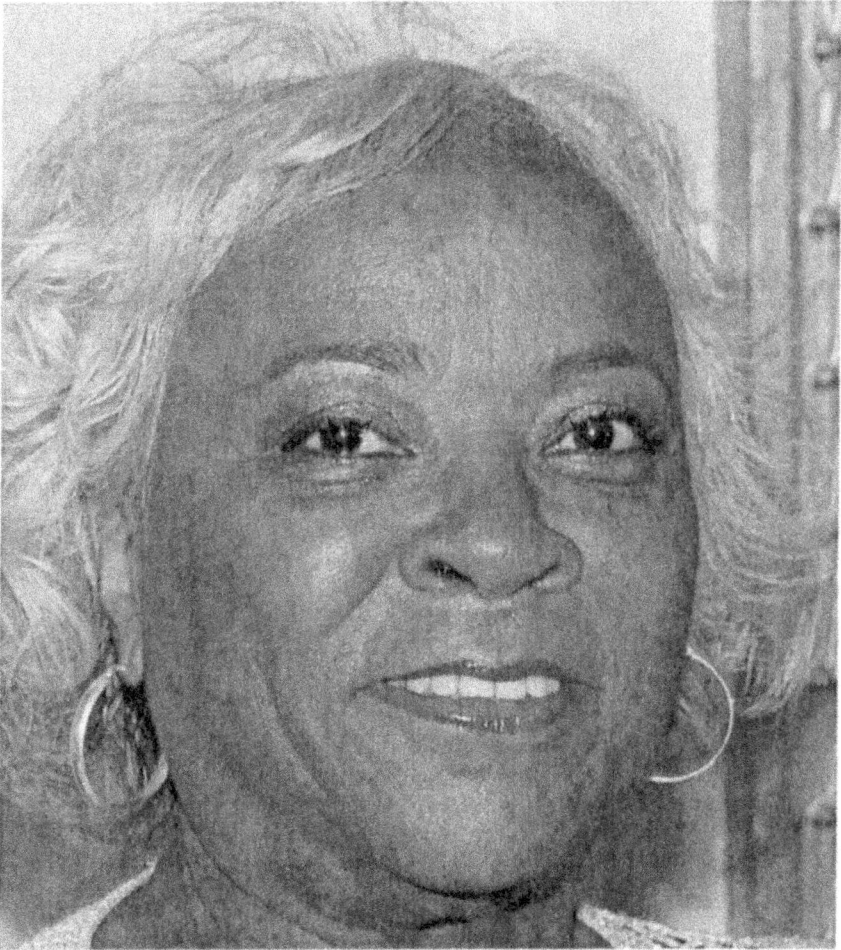

Never use old relaxers make sure they are fresh. If you smell a strong scent that generally indicates an unsanitary or damaging product. Make sure the stylist is cleaning the scissors, razors, clippers, and combs. If you allow bad habits to happen then the hair stylist will probably get worse. State Board will visit the salon twice a year so watch how your stylist makes those corrections. If the stylist is willing to make improvements for the State Board, then why not for you?

THE GOLDEN GIRLS AND THEIR HAIR

Now it is time for the right season, and it is the season for the Golden Girls. They wear all colors, black, brown, gray, red, and a mixture of highlights. I have had seasoned clients with the most beautiful gray hair and it is a blessing from God! Now, how do you keep the gray shiny and bright? First, what causes the gray not to shine? It can have a lot to do with smoking, medication, and the products that you put in your hair. Grays can be rekindled by using rinses, shampoos, and conditioners. All of these products will pull the green and yellow discoloration out. Shimmering Lights is wonderful to use as well. It has a purple tint so don't over use it. Over heating the hair can change the gray to a yellowish tint, so try setting the hair before attempting to curl the hair.

As you mature, hair thinning may occur. Make sure it is not due to bad hair habits. Alert your hair stylist and make sure that you get the proper treatments. Sit under the dryer at least twice a month with a reconstructor conditioner. Keep a clean cut or clean ends. Short hair styles often look more elegant on mature ladies. A short hair cut can save you time, especially if you can't spend as much time in the salon. Wear a layered bob, or a tapered hair cut that frames your face perfectly. Long hair can look wonderful for those who prefer it, and have maintained long healthy hair over the years. Taking hair vitamins will also strengthen the hair and are recommended if you are noticing hair loss. Log on to the www.discoveryhealth.com, and consult your doctor to make sure that the product will not interfere with your medication. Some medications will cause hair loss despite the efforts you make to avoid hair loss. Consult with your doctor and discuss other medications that can be substituted to avoid continuous hair loss. Vitamin C has been a wonderful substance for my clients.

As you mature, be conscious of how frequently you color your hair. Excessive coloring is particularly harmful for mature hair. Some mature clients can't wear black hair if dark circles have developed under or around their eyes. The dark hair only brings attention to the dark circles. Features will change the more you mature, so try to wear a hair style and color that will enhance you. Gray hair doesn't look good on everyone especially if the hair is too thin or damaged. Some clients look tired and worn out, while others look vibrant and renewed with gray hair. Try on some wigs to see what color or style looks great on you. Take a picture to see if your hair stylist can give you that look you desire.

Who can properly do your hair as a golden girl; my advice is to find someone who has the patience and time. As you mature, sitting in the salon is the last thing you would want to do. Try to be the first client, and make sure your hair stylist has a good sense of time. If you can't make it to the salon then ask your hair stylist to order some products for you to use at home. There are some hair stylists who make house calls if you're unable to physically leave the house, see if they can make a house call.

Now that you have decided to wear a wig then please wear a stylish one that has body and looks fabulous. Keep a couple of 100% human hair wigs, and clean them like you would do your own hair. Your hair stylist can cut them to fit your head. Human hair can be set as well. Take your wig off around the house so that your hair can breathe. Wearing them all the time may result in hair loss. Make sure you still keep your hair shampooed, and conditioned. Oil your scalp with vitamin A, D and E oil.

Golden Girls, I love you! Enjoy your years by putting your make up on and polishing your nails. Now don't forget to wear your hair fabulous and free. I have seen some ladies who have the right recipe for life; they look so breath taking. There are a few Golden Girls that I have had the pleasure of styling their hair or I have seen them in the community. I refer to then as HOLLYWOOD. If you need a consultation, log on to, www.thehealthyhair.com.

Barbering

Men have grown into loving hair care just like women. The times have changed. They are getting, cuts, shaves, facials, manicures, pedicures, colors, and massages. Nioxin also makes a lot of products that will

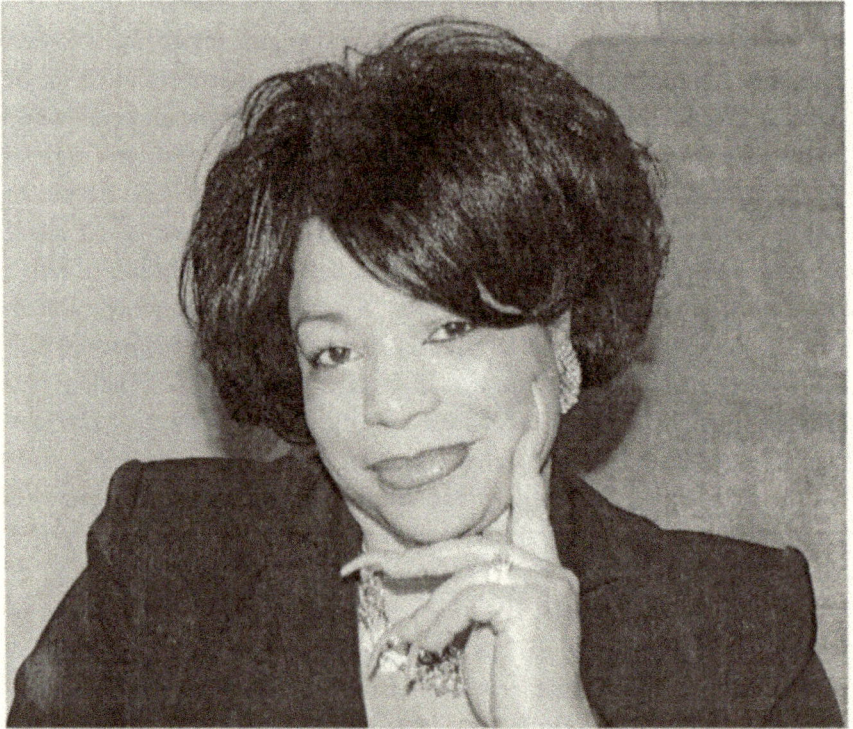

decrease baldness. You can still remain masculine and get the personal touch, remember you deserve it!

I interviewed Bryan Caple, a barber at Kreativ Kutz in Memphis TN. Bryan makes customized hair brushes that will promote healthy hair texture. I asked Bryan what separates him from other barbers and he explained, "The way I keep my tools and chair bacteria free." Before each hair cut he cleans each blade. Clients keep coming back, because of his precision cutting and sanitary habits. Razor bumps come from unclean clippers and blades that cut too close. Bryan explains, "Barbers must clean their brushes after each use, by rinsing with warm water and barbercide." He places a special touch by cleaning his chair to assure that each client will be free from any bacteria infection. H42 is also used to clean his blades; this assures that none of his clients will get any disease, or infection. Bryan emphasized that once a pathogenic bacteria enters into the hair follicle it can cause infection and swelling. Once this occurs then the hair shaft may start to curl under the damaged surface. This will and can irritate the skin. Medications and specially formulated creams can kill the bacteria.

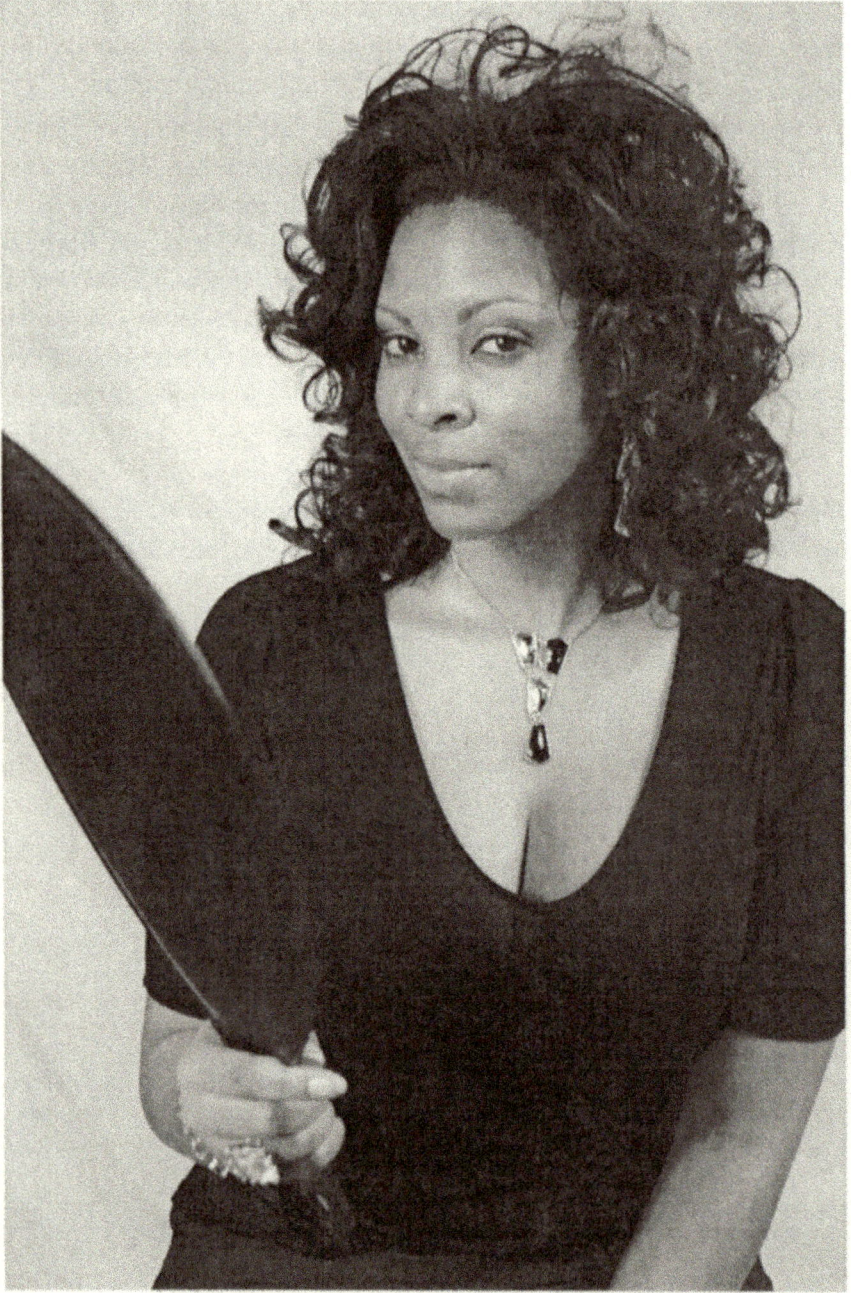

Chapter Thirteen
How To Get The Sexy Back In Your Hair!

===

SEXY HAIR IS IN everyone, so breathe in and out and shout out loud, I BROUGHT SEXY BACK INTO MY HAIR! Calling all hair dos short, medium, long, curly, wavy, straight, and all textures. Love your hair, you can't wear every hair style so wear the best style for you, this will bring out the best in you! No one can take that from you whatever your signature style is. Let your hair blow in the wind, and work it like you're a runway model. I suggest you begin by looking at your face and how it is structured then research for different hair do's. For fun go to a wig store and see if you can find your style, look in hair books, or even on the web. Make whatever style you choose sexy. Sexy hair has to be healthy so shampoo your hair and condition it, and clean those ends up! Color can be fun as well and add some pizzazz to your new look. I love all lengths, the bob can be cute in any length, it goes back in time, and it still has remained popular. You can make it long or medium; you can add layers for volume. If you go short then keep it jazzy not boring. Spike it or flat iron it or curl it just right! The cut is the key, so find the right stylist who can master the perfect cut. If you're looking for the set style for a special occasion then make sure it is elegant and classy for the after five affair. I love styling hair for weddings and any special occasion.

For years I have mastered elegant hair dos, my client's can usually wear anything because I practice healthy hair. I have fulfilled mostly all of their fantasy hair styles. I am the one stop shop, now this ego is just as confident on their hair. I have earned the right, I put the hard work into the business for twenty years, and I love it! I love every one of my clients they encourage me to push to higher learning. The biggest thing I have earned with each of my client's is TRUST! Not every stylist can say that. Lord knows I appreciate them, because this is a hustle kind of business not every stylist survives in the hair business.

As for words of wisdom to the new hair stylist, connect with your clients. Find another career if you hate the public, working for the public is not easy. I sometimes run out of fuel, and I have to regroup, clients are smart so watch the attitude! Remember they are your bread and butter, and when you go home leave work at work, and the same vice versa.

Hair can be fun so look sexy in your hair and you'll get that new job, or man, or woman, or anything you can dream of! My famous quote has been success begins with the hair! Hair is alive so treat it that way, don't weigh it down with heavy oils or clog it up with too much spritz, which can dry out the hair. Educate yourselves learn what works and what doesn't.

If you can't afford to go to the hair stylist every week then go every two weeks. If that is not affordable, try to at least visit every six weeks and consult with your hair stylist to get the same products at home ordered for maintenance care. It doesn't help to use cheap products at home and expensive products at the salon, which defeats the purpose. Love yourself enough to stop spending hundreds or thousands of dollars on purses, wardrobes and only a few dollars on your hair. Your hair can affect your mood and self esteem. Now when your hair is full of life you can walk in a room and be recognized and be confident in yourself.

Keep in mind that the following are important ingredients to look for in products:

+ Biotin D & C
+ Hydrolyzed Keratin Protein
+ Animal Protein
+ Protein
+ Deionized Water

- Propylene Glycol
- Soybean Oil
- Glycerin Stearate
- Mineral Oil
- Wheat Protein
- Dimethicone
- Sugar cane
- Java Oil

These ingredients strengthen the hair and produce moisture. Wheat protein, animal protein, biotin D&C, and dimethicone have agents that tighten the hair shaft and control hair loss. The hair care system that I provide for my clients, contain the above ingredients that have proven results for strengthening hair, promoting hair growth, and adding body.

Try taking pictures of your different hair styles and always see what looks classy and what needs to stay in the past. Your hair can speak to you it will make a quiet popping sound when it is breaking, it will squeak when it is too dry, or it will fall quietly on your shoulders to alarm you that more hair might be leaving you soon. So don't ignore these sounds, remember to keep your hair healthy, and get your sexy back, you deserve it!

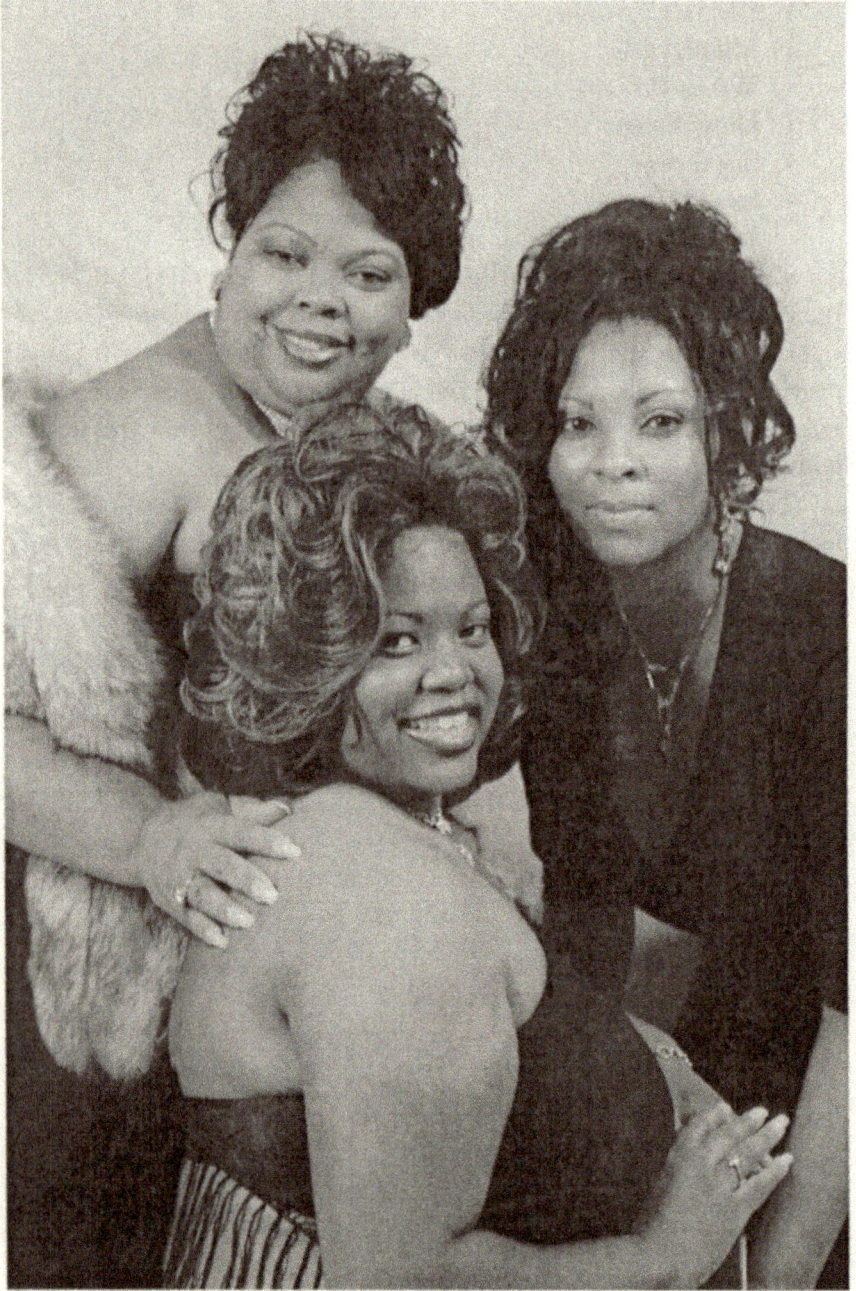

Q & A

The guessing game is over! The following is a list of the most frequently asked questions concerning hair. In addition, you will find a few references, concerning hair products, vitamins, beauty tips, and much more.

Q: Can I get a perm and a chemical color at the same time?

A: Definitely NO. Two chemicals processes at the same time will result in hair loss. Wait two to three weeks to allow the hair to strengthen following a chemical treatment.

Q: Will pure protein damage my hair if I use it weekly?

A: Yes pure protein is only necessary to use if shedding is occurring. When shedding is no longer a problem and the hair strands are strong, discontinue use of protein, to avoid protein damage.

Q: Can my child get a perm before the age of five?

A: Yes, but I would recommend that you try a very mild relaxer, no lye, or a texturizer.

Q: How often should you keep your ends clipped?

A: It depends on the client and their at home habits. If your hair is healthy then every four weeks, if your hair is damaged then clipping the ends every two to three weeks maybe beneficial. Remember clipping the ends is not extreme cutting; therefore, it will not change the length of your hair if done properly.

Q: What is the best pillow case to sleep on?

A: Any high thread count 100% cotton, or a high quality satin pillow case. High thread counts are 350-600.

Q: If I am wearing a weave pony tail, how long can I wear it before it becomes damaging?

A: The weight of the weave pony tail is too heavy to wear over a long period of time. Thinning may occur at the top of your crown if you begin wearing it over a period of months.

Q: What can help my hair and scalp if dryness occurs?

A: Hot oil treatments, moisturizing conditioners, and vitamin scalp oils.

Q: When getting a chemical color, what volume is too high and damaging to apply and mix with the color application?

A: Of course, 30 to 40 volumes are too damaging to use, the hair takes time to break down and the chemical can severely give the hair long term hair lose. Boosters are too strong as well especially on fine, dry hair, or long hair.

Q: Is it possible to experience hair loss while sleeping?

A: Yes the brain is a weight, and if you sleep on the same side every night you may see thinning in that area. What you put on your head matters. Make sure you clean any items that you may use to secure your hair. Satin and 100% cotton caps are very safe. Other items may pull the hair strands and snap off the hair.

Q: If I am wearing dreads in my hair, will my hair thin out?

A: Yes, if you do not maintain them. Some people do not keep them refreshed and the weight of the dread pulls the hair attached and causes the hair to thin. Once you decide to cut them off, then you have to start all over and treat the hair to promote growth.

Q: Should I pull the relaxer throughout my hair every time I get a touch up?

A: No, that will result in over processing. The hair will thin out and the texture will change. The only exception is after years of relaxing, when the hair starts to revert at the mid section to the ends, then you may have to perform a virgin perm or relaxer.

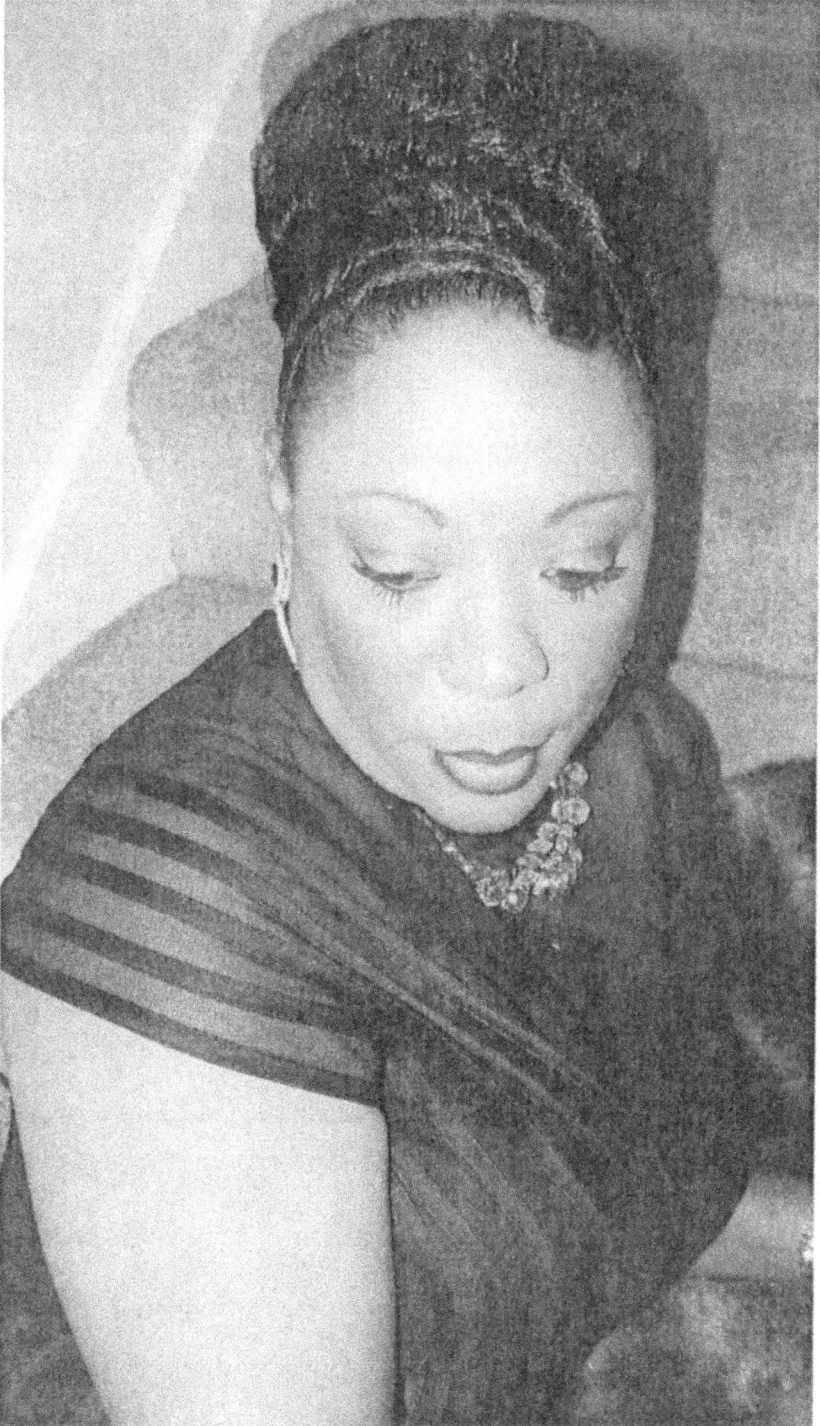

Q: Will I experience hair loss, if I wear my weave or wig too long.?

A: Yes, the wigs and weaves can be too heavy for the hair, and hair has to breathe.

Q: If my hair is gray what can I put in my hair to get the green or yellow out?

A: Shimmering Lights is a conditioner and shampoo that will give the hair a clear gray look. Hair rinses for gray hair have been successful, and they are safe. Putting a protector conditioner on the hair will shield the hair from changing colors.

Q: Will drinking water help my hair grow?

A: Drinking water will keep the hair healthy and strong. Dryness can occur in the scalp and hair strand if you fail to drink adequate amounts of water.

Q: Once I reach the age of sixty will my hair start to fall out due to maturing?

A: No, only if you start bad habits with your hair. Hair loss may occur due to genetics. Staying healthy and exercising will keep your hair on the right track. If illness occurs, then check with your doctor to see if your medication has any side effects that will cause hair loss.

Q: Can I get a hair rinse when I get a relaxer?

A: Yes this particular color process is a non- chemical treatment.

Q: Will hair gels and holding sprays cause my hair to become damaged over a period of time?

A: Yes, if you over use them. Anything with alcohol can be damaging if you don't apply hair oil to your hair.

Q: Is olive oil and aloe good for my hair?

A: Yes, they are full of vitamins and minerals, plus they add moisture to the hair.

Q: If I am going to the barber shop weekly and I am wearing a hat every day, will my hair thin out?

A: Over a period of time your hair will thin out. The scalp needs to breathe, and the hat is preventing the hair growth. Men still need hair care; my male customers still receive hair treatments.

Q: Can everyone in the house use the same comb and brush?

A: Everyone should have their own comb and brush. Sharing hair accessories, combs and brushes can spread dandruff and other skin conditions. You would never share your toothbrush; therefore, you should never share your hairbrush. Such items should be considered personal to promote healthy hair. If you must share, make sure you use barbercide to clean the comb and brush after each use.

Q: What are the best vitamins for my hair and nails?

A: Nioxin has a wonderful vitamin, Recharging Complex. This vitamin has a balanced nutritional supplementation, and will strengthen your hair and nails. It has been known for improving the appearance of the skin as well.

Vitamin Life Spray, has a Pre-Natal spray vitamin that targets straight to your system by misting it directly in your mouth. This vitamin is just not for pregnant women. The benefits are great because it also strengthens the hair and nails. www.lifesprayvitamins.net.

Q: What can I use on my scalp for thinning and balding areas that is excessive?

A: Nioxin took the time to create the Follicle Booster, that is for people who have noticeable thinning, and balding areas. This product is applied directly to the scalp only. Apply twice a day, morning, and at night.

<u>(References to find products, web sites, and health and beauty aid.)</u>

Looking for a master healthy hair braider, contact Brinetta D. Carlton. Whether you desire, braids, sisterlocks, weaves and much more, she can consult you on what's best for you. Give her a call, 901-949-2423, or e-mail, brinetta2@gmail.com www.lifesprayvitamins.net, for a healthier you from A-Z......

www.ardysslife.com/angelanewlook, vitamins, body shapers, Levive, Noni, weight loss, and much more...........

www.thehealthyhair.com, where you will be able to purchase consultation packages, and see my latest hair styles, and educate yourself on more hair care. Order your books online through www.amazon.com and enjoy all my fiction, and non fiction books.......

www.emmaculatecomplexion.com, Specializing in body wraps, skin care, and make up artistry, ask for Tiffany Ross, 901-474-9958

www.pillowpockets.com, e-mail, sheilalester@jaylesterandcompany.com, Enjoy a high thread count satin pillow case, custom made colors available........

Alopecia treatments, balding treatments, Itchy scalp treatment, www.scalpicin.com

How to stop baldness, www.smartorganicproducts.com/baldness

Looking for more healthy hair tips check out, www.discoveryhealth.com

Need to know what products work, e-mail, angela@thehealthyhair.com

Need to correct your baldness, hair and scalp check out, www.nioxin.com,

Looking for more answers concerning beauty and hair tips, then listen in to our radio show, **"LET'S TALK HAIR",** wear you can call in on any hair care question. Log on to www.thehealthyhair.com, or www.letstalkhealthyhair.com, or www.blogtalkradio.com.

Looking to build a **BIG RESIDUAL CLIENTELE,** then ask me how, e-mail, angela@thehealthyhair.com

Xs Quizit Lotions Candles, has candles that melts into a silky lotion, smell the enticing aroma, contact, Likisha Nichols, 501-804-8030. www.xlcandles.com

Special Thanks!

Perry C. Brown, photographer, Artistic Impression, 901-314-9828, or 1800-991-3032 perry_brownsr@yahoo.com

Michael Owens photographer, contact information www.londonsbridge. smugmug.com

Tiffany Harrison, makeup artist, contact information, 901-573-4792

Thanks to Alberta Nibely, salon owner (Concepts 2000 Beauty and Barbering) Memphis Tennessee 38108

Thanks to Kimberly William Greer, hair stylist and personal stylist for the Food Network show *Down Home with the Neely's*, and *Road Tasted with the Neely's*. Contact information, 901-289-0257

Thanks to Bryan Caple, barber, at Kreativ Kutz in Memphis Tennessee. Bryan custom makes hair brushes just for each client, give him a call at 901-463-8314

Thanks so much to all my hair models, Adrienne H. Jackson, April Miller, Cassandra Jackson, Crystal Howard, Johnnie O Ijames, Mlidred Ashford, Raven, Rosie Bond, Sauna Tate, Shanance Jones, Raven Hinton, Valinus Rodgers, and Victoria Crenshaw

Angela Hughes Brown has paid her dues in this billion dollar industry. She has mastered her way to the top educating so many people on how to get to know their hair. Not only is it her career it is also her true talent crafted by trial an error. She is an author, inventor, motivational speaker, and hair stylist consultant. She has recently become a member of Toast Masters, to improve her speaking skills, she loves to connect with her audience, and pull them in the room. When she speaks about hair she goes into another world, and nothing else seems to matter. Angela H. Brown is a hair and scalp specialist for Nioxin a well known hair and scalp product line. God has truly blessed her career. Angela H. Brown is on the move and finally following all of her dreams. She has no plans on slowing down! Stay tuned for her new DVD, HOW TO GET THE SEXY BACK IN YOUR HAIR. This is hands on techniques for all occasions. Angela H. Brown has launched her radio show "LET'S TALK HAIR", were callers can call in and ask any hair care questions. She also welcomes any guest to net work their business and help educate others on how to keep their hair, body, and total up scale healthy look. Angela H. Brown encourages everyone to get on board to rekindle their dreams, because she is in a **"YES WE CAN MOOD"**!

How To Get The Healthy Back In Your Hair, Will.........

1. This book will educate you on the do's and don'ts.
2. Learn hair tips.
3. How to choose the right hair stylist.
4. Motivate you on how to look sexy in your hair.
5. When to leave your hair stylist.
6. What you're paying for.
7. Budget idea's for your hair.
8. Exciting healthy techniques.

www.ingramcontent.com/pod-product-compliance
Lightning Source LLC
Chambersburg PA
CBHW022127280326
41933CB00007B/579